The
SOUNDS
Of The
NORMAL HEART

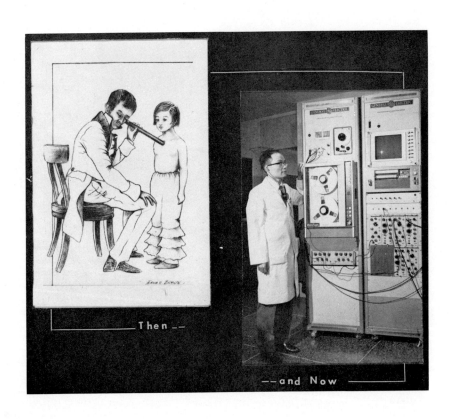

Then --

--and Now

The
SOUNDS
Of The
NORMAL HEART

By

ALDO A. LUISADA, M.D.

Professor of Medicine and Professor of Physiology and Biophysics
The Chicago Medical School, University of Health Sciences
Attending Cardiologist, Mount Sinai Hospital Medical Center
Chicago, Illinois

WARREN H. GREEN, INC.
St. Louis, Missouri, U.S.A.

iii

Published by

WARREN H. GREEN, INC.
10 South Brentwood Boulevard
Saint Louis, Missouri 63105, U. S. A.

Library of Congress Catalog Card Number 78-176172

Printed in the United States of America

To little Andrea

Preface

This book is based on thirty years of experience with phonocardiography.

Apart from several publications on the subject, two previous books by the author (*Heart,* 1949 and 1954, and *Heart Beat,* 1953) contained numerous phonocardiographic documents. The first treatise correlated phonocardiographic data with other clinical evidence of heart disease; the second compared phonocardiography with other graphic methods used in the study of cardiac patients. Another book by the author and Liu (*Cardiac Pressures and Pulses,* 1956; later *Intracardiac Phenomena,* 1958) was primarily devoted to the methods of cardiac catheterization and contained several chapters devoted to intracardiac phonocardiography. Finally, the book *From Auscultation to Phonocardiography* (1965) correlated the two aspects of the method, the physiologic and the technical. This new book represents a further step, and it is hoped that it will contribute to the training of physicians and to an enrichment of their knowledge.

The names of two of the author's coworkers, Drs. Zalter and MacCanon deserve special mention for their long collaborration and their original contributions to problems of phonocardiography. The technical help of J. Morris and I. Harvey has been invaluable for the physiologic studies.

Numerous researchers have worked in the author's laboratory on problems of phonocardiography. Their names should be mentioned because of their original contributions and because they brought the experience of many countries as well as their youthful enthusiasm. In order of date, they are: H. Mautner, L. Weisz, L. Wolff, F. Romano, M. Roitman, L. Pérez Montes, F. Mendoza, J. Torre, G. Magri, S. Contro, A. B. Zilli, M. Haring, L. Cardi, C. Aravanis, L. Richmond, G. Gamna, E. Jona, C. K. Liu, J. Bendezú-Prieto, M. R. Testelli, C. Friedland, A. Jacono, J. Szatkowski, G. Di Bartolo, D. Nuñez-Dey, J. P. Constantino, T. Inoue, R. Reich, T. Mori, M. Katz, F. Arevalo, E. Meyer, S. J. Slodki, T. Sakamoto, R. Kusukawa, B. Argano, J. Oravetz, H. Kurz, S. Wissner, B. Placik, M. Worthen, L. Feigen, and A. Sakai.

This book was prepared during tenure of Training Grant HE-5002 of the National Heart Institute, U. S. Public Health Service.

Editorial considerations have induced the author to divide the material in two parts. This book *(The Sounds of the Normal Heart)* represents the first part. Another book *(The Sounds of the Diseased Heart)* will appear one year later.

I would like to thank Ms. James W. Morris and Ivan Harvey for their valuable collaboration to animal experiments and Mrs. Dorothy M. Lewis for the preparation of the manuscript.

A. A. L.

CONTENTS

PART V — TECHNICAL ASPECTS OF PHONOCARDIOGRAPHY

PART VI — ROUTINE PHONOCARDIOGRAPHIC STUDY

PART VII — THE NORMAL VIBRATORY PHENOMENON OF THE
PRECORDIUM

The
SOUNDS
Of The
NORMAL HEART

Part I
PRELIMINARY

Chapter 1

The Problem

CLASSIC AUSCULTATION was developed over a century ago at a time when physiologic knowledge was poor and hemodynamic studies in man were not possible. Most of the basic data were obtained by listening to hearts, noting the abnormalities of sound, and then correlating them with autopsy findings. This procedure yielded notable results in spite of the fact that many patients either were never autopsied or died several years after a certain sound or murmur was noted.

Most of the important data of clinical auscultation were known and correctly evaluated nearly a century ago, at the time of Potain. Splitting of the second sound; triple rhythms; the opening snap, the characteristic rumbling rhythm of mitral stenosis; the harsh systolic murmur of aortic or pulmonary valvular stenosis; the blowing, soft diastolic murmur of aortic or pulmonary insufficiency; and the blowing systolic murmur of mitral or tricuspid insufficiency were correctly evaluated before the end of last century. These data then became part of a "classic" body of knowledge, and this rendered their revision a difficult and slow process. In spite of wide acceptance, dissatisfaction with current teaching was often noted among physicians because frequently the data that they obtained did not agree with the "classic" interpretation.

The slow revision of auscultation in the last few decades can be attributed to these reasons: (1) the acumen and enthusiasm of the clinicians who reaped an early harvest in a fertile field; (2) the limitations of the auditory system of man and of physical diagnosis in general; (3) the reluctance of physicians to change their beliefs, which had been firmly ingrained in their mind during their period of training.

Following great developments of cardiovascular physiology in the years between 1910 and 1940, catheterization in man opened a new possibility by allowing the cardiologist, through exact hemodynamic evaluation, not only to confirm a diagnosis during life but also to quantitate the severity of a cardiac dysfunction —be this the result of a shunt, a valvular lesion, a metabolic disturbance, or myocardial weakness.

Along with cardiac catheterization, phonocardiography has become a more exact art. It gives us a permanent record of auscultatory findings, corrects auditory illusions, allows us to check contradictory statements, and reveals facts undisclosed by the human ear—an imperfect physical system.

A further stage, intracardiac phonocardiography, results from the combination of two methods. This new procedure, used in both patients and experimental animals, has added important information, particularly in regard to the timing of sounds and to the site of origin of sounds and murmurs. Further knowledge has been obtained by high speed cineangiocardiographic studies, by study of the cardiac valves during open heart procedures, and by study of sounds created by artificial heart valves.

Old viewpoints unfortunately tend to be perpetuated and hamper changes that are overdue. Classic auscultation should be continuously revised by checking each statement with new accurate data and more complete knowledge.

Work done in our laboratory has led to several contributions that allow us to better interpret sound recordings and extract greater information from them.

The motion of the heart, transmitted to the chest wall, results in a complex *vibratory phenomenon*. The heart sounds and murmurs are but a part of this vibration, which is artificially selected by either the human ear or the phonocardiography. Another part of this phenomenon is recorded by the low-frequency tracings, and is grossly appreciated by inspection and palpation.

The *auditory system of man* is not ideally suited for cardiac auscultation. Knowledge of its limitations explains some of the pitfalls of auscultation and certain unavoidable discrepancies between clinical impressions and objective data.

In order to obtain satisfactory tracings, the phonocardiograph makes use of *filters* that select the desired frequency band to be recorded. Certain cardiac phenomena acquire particular emphasis in the lower whereas others need to be studied in the higher frequency bands.

A revision of the *areas of asucultation* has been suggested by the author correlating these areas with the actual sound phenomena found within the various cardiac chambers and large vessels as well as with sounds recorded over such areas.

Physicians and investigators should keep an open mind in regards to auscultation, a field that is undergoing growing pains.

The studies of the last twenty years have gradually changed the scope and instrumentation of phonocardiography. This can be defined at present as the method of recording all vibrations of the precordium.* As such, it is different from auscultation because: (1) it has a greater scope; (2) it is not bound by the limitations of the auditory system with its selective emphasis of certain bands, its distortion of certain sounds, and its inability to hear other sounds; (3) it may apply itself to a separate study of different vibratory aspects in different frequency bands; (4) it permits accurate timing of the cardiac sounds, and (5) it preserves a permanent document.

Phonocardiography has been further developed through the use of *magnetic tape recorders*. These enable us to transmit the tracing by telephone, to study it by means of computers, to record it either unfiltered or through filters, and finally to study it visually with the help of an oscilloscope. The latter is extremely helpful for teaching auscultation because it adds a new dimen-

---

*Our definition is far more comprehensive than an older one advocated by clinical cardiologists, which restricted phonocardiography to the recording of clinically audible vibrations. As shown in Chapter 4, this definition might lead to a change in name, so that the method could be called *acousticardiography* or *mechanocardiography*.

sion by integrating the data of auscultation (ear) with those supplied by vision (eye).

It is often forgotten that some of the difficulties of auscultation are the result of two shortcomings; one is the lack of an accurate timer, the other is the impossibility of slowing down sounds that follow each other with great rapidity. Both are remedied by phonocardiography, which spreads the vibrations through the high speed of the recording film and simultaneously records other tracings for "timing."

A frequent source of controversy arises from the fact that an observer can hear a certain sound or murmur on a certain day whereas others cannot hear it either on the same day or on subsequent days. This can result from different auditory thresholds, changing conditions of cardiodynamics, or progression of pathologic phenomena. It can be remedied by immediate recording of the phenomena on a tape or on a phonocardiographic film.

For all the enumerated reasons, phonocardiography, if the method is correctly applied through adequate instrumentation and the tracings are correctly interpreted by a trained observer, has a definite superiority over auscultation. This fact should be recognized without embarrassment by clinical cardiologists and without undue proudness by specialists of phonocardiography. Autopsy findings have been considered more reliable than clinical impressions for centuries; this does not involve a diminution in the stature of the clinician.

Therefore, phonocardiography should take its place next to auscultation, which it enriches, guides, and checks by means of a fruitful collaboration.

Chapter 2

Historical Developments of
Auscultation and Phonocardiography

THE FIRST mention of "auscultation" can be found in Ebers' papyrus from ancient Egypt. However, that text states that the physician should "listen" to the heart by applying his fingers to the anterior chest wall. Therefore, such instruction pertains to palpation, not to auscultation.

It is likely that for many centuries the physicians applied their ear to the precordium of patients and felt an impulse while they heard certain sounds. However, there is no record of their observations.

W. Harvey (1628) stated that "the heart is the cause of an audible impulse" but his observation was met with denial and skepticism.

Corvisart and Bayle stated that they applied their ear to the chest in order to hear the sounds of the heart but Laennec denied that they did actually perform the act of listening.

Laennec (1781-1826), therefore, was the first who, not only applied his ear to the chest in order to listen to the sounds of the heart (direct or immediate auscultation), but also invented the stethoscope (indirect or mediate auscultation). He also described the first and second sounds, the triple rhythms, and most murmurs. Inadequate physiologic knowledge of the time led to

9

a faulty interpretation of the heart sounds. This was corrected, however, by the middle of the 19th century.

The observations of Hope, Bouillaud, Gendrin, Potain, Corrigan, Traube, Bramwell, Flint, DaCosta, Duroziez, Mackenzie, Skoda, and many others established the fundamental bases of cardiac auscultation.

In the first quarter of the 20th century, Vaquez, Huchard, Gallavardin, Laubry, Lian, Lutembacher, and Routier in France; Martini and Weber in Germany; Cardarelli, Castellino, Pezzi and Frugoni in Italy; Thayer, S. A. Levine, Kerr, and P. D. White in the United States contributed valuable data in regard to auscultation. Subsequent contributions are so intimately connected with phonocardiographic studies that they cannot be easily separated from the latter.

The first recording of heart sounds was made by Huerthle (1895), who connected a microphone to an inductorium, the secondary coil of which stimulated a nerve-muscle preparation of a frog. At about the same time, Einthoven recorded phonocardiograms, first by means of a capillary electrometer, and then with a string galvanometer. He was followed by Th. Lewis, who recorded clinical phonocardiograms by means of a string galvanometer. Direct phonocardiograms were subsequently recorded by O. Frank with his segment capsule. A modification of Frank's capsule was described by Wiggers, and was used by Orias and Braun-Menéndez for recording heart sounds and murmurs from the chest wall. The first monograph of phonocardiography was published by O. Weiss in 1909.

Subsequent developments resulted from the development of the vacuum tube, which made electronic amplification possible.

The best known texts* or phonocardiography were written by Orias and Braun-Menéndez, 1937 and 1939; (Lian, Minot, and Welti, 1941) ; Weber, 1944; (Levine and Harvey, 1949) ; Calo, 1950; Schmidt-Voigt, 1951; Luisada, 1953; (Butterworth et al., 1955) ; Holldack and Wolf, 1956; Weber, 1956; (Ravin, 1958) ; McKusick, 1958; Heintzen, 1960; Ueda, Kaito, and Sakamoto, 1963; Luisada, 1965; Günther, 1969.

*Authors in parentheses wrote primarily from the point of view of auscultation, while phonocardiographic data were included mainly for the purpose of documentation or demonstration.

Among the significant studies of the last thirty years are the following:

1. Studies of Schuetz in Germany on the origin of heart sounds and on cardiodynamics (1929-1934).
2. Clinical studies of Wolferth and Margolies in Philadelphia (1933-1935).
3. Studies of Orias and Braun-Menéndez in Buenos Aires (1935-1939).
4. Studies of Mannheimer in Sweden (calibrated phonocardiography) (1939-1941).
5. Studies of Rappaport and Sprague in Boston (laws of auscultation; linear, stethoscopic, and logarithmic phonocardiography) (1940-1942).
6. Technical studies of Maass and Weber in Germany that led to better construction of phonocardiographs, and clinical studies of Holldack with such equipment (1952-1956).
7. Clinical studies of Leatham in Great Britain with medium high-frequency phonocardiograms resulting in a better knowledge of the heart sounds (1950-1955).
8. Studies of Luisada, Zalter, and co-workers in Chicago, who re-examined the bases of phonocardiography, built an experimental phonocardiograph, and recorded high-frequency tracings in clinical cases (1959-1961).
10. Studies of Eddleman in Birmingham and of Dimond and co-workers in La Jolla with ultralow frequency tracings of the precordium (1953-1963).
11. Experimental studies of Luisada, MacCanon, and co-workers in Chicago on the hemodynamic correlates of the heart sounds (1961-1970). Application of the experimental data to clinical studies.
12. Studies of Luisada, MacCanon, and Feigen in Chicago resulting in the construction of a new calibrated phonocardiograph (1969-1970) with tape recording, band pass filtration, and single or double differentiation of the output of a displacement microphone.

The following books represent the main landmarks of phonocardiography:

Orias, O., and Braun-Menéndez, E.: *The Heart Sounds in Normal and Pathological Conditions,* London, 1939, Oxford University Press.

Lian, C., Minot, G., and Welti, J. J.: *Phonocardiographie, Auscultation Collective,* Paris, 1941, Masson & Cie.

Weber, A.: *Herzschallregistrierung,* Darmstadt, 1944, Dietrich Steinkopff.

Levine, S., and Harvey, W. P.: *Clinical Auscultation of the Heart,* Philadelphia, 1949, W. B. Saunders Co.

Calo, A.: *Les Bruits du Coeur et des Vaisseaux,* Paris, 1950, Masson & Cie.

Schmidt-Voigt, J.: *Herzschalldiagnostik in Klink und Praxis,* Stuttgart, 1951, Georg Thieme Verlag.

Luisada, A. A.: *The Heart Beat,* New York, 1953, Paul B. Hoeber, Inc.

Butterworth, J. S., Chassin, M. R., and McGrath, R.: *Cardiac Auscultation,* New York, 1955, Grune & Stratton, Inc.

Holldack, K. and Wolf, D.: *Atlas und Kurzgefasstes Lehrbuch der Phonokardiographie und Verwandter Untersuchungsmethoden.* Stuttgart, 1956, Georg Thieme Verlag.

McKusick, V. A.: *Cardiovascular Sound in Health and Disease,* Baltimore, 1958, Williams & Wilkins Co.

Ravin, A.: *Auscultation of the Heart,* Chicago, 1958, Year Book Medical Publishers, Inc.

Heintzen, P.: *Quantitative Phonokardiographie,* Stuttgart, 1960, Georg Thieme Verlag.

Ueda, H., Kaito, G., and Sakamoto, T.: *Clinical Phonocardiography* (Japanese), Tokyo, 1963, Nanzando.

Segal, B. L., Likoff, W., and Moyer, J. H.: *The Theory and Practice of Auscultation,* Philadelphia, 1964, F. A. Davis Co.

Luisada, A. A.: *From Auscultation to Phonocardiography,* St. Louis, 1965, Mosby.

Guenther, K. H.: *Vergleichende Extrakardiale und Intrakardiale Phonocardiographie,* Berlin, 1969, Akademie Verlag.

Chapter 3

Definitions

THE FOLLOWING statements and definitions will be discussed in Parts II, III, and IV.

1. *Sounds* are mechanical vibrations in air having frequencies between 20 and 16,000 cycles per second and a magnitude that is sufficient to excite the average auditory system of man.

2. *Acoustic phenomena* are wave-like, mechanical vibrations of any frequency and magnitude. Therefore, they may be either audible or inaudible.

3. The heart generates *acoustic vibrations* of different duration and frequency. A *click* (or *snap* or *knock*) is a sound of relatively high frequency and very short duration. A *heart sound* is a group of mixed vibrations of short duration. A *murmur* is a group of mixed vibrations of long duration. Some of these acoustic phenomena are either below audibility or in a range where audition is poor.

4. The *auscultatory and phonocardiographic areas of the precordium* are partly overlapping and vary in location and extension from individual to individual. None of them allows exclusive identification of a sound or murmur.

5. The heart sounds are *not* caused by clapping of the valve leaflets. They are only partly caused by valve tension. The *first heart sound* is caused by ventricular contraction, and the major portion of its energy derives from an oscillation of a

closely coupled "cardiohemic" system composed of the left ventricular blood and its surrounding structures. The *second heart sound* is caused by kinetic changes of the arterial blood as a result of cessation of ventricular contraction, the major portion of its energy deriving from the arterial walls and the blood.

Valve function is important for the *timing* of sounds because ventricular and arterial tensions require prior valve closure or opening.

6. Most of the so-called "valve" snaps or clicks originate in the cardiac chambers and *not* in the valves themselves with the exception of the clicks caused by artificial valves.

7. *Phonocardiography* is a method that provides visual observation, graphic recording, storage and analysis of information regarding the acoustic phenomena caused by the cardiac action, whether audible or not.

8. *Mechanocardiography* is a method that provides visual observation, graphic recording, storage, and analysis of information regarding the ultra-low motions of the precordium, as well as the arterial and venous pulses.

Part II

PHYSICS OF SOUND

PHYSIOLOGY OF SOUND PERCEPTION

Chapter 4

Sound and Acoustics

THERE IS NO general agreement about the definition of the term "sound," this word having been used with either a physical or physiologic connotation. The following definitions have been suggested by Randall.

Acoustics is that branch of physics which deals with the generation of mechanical vibrations of any frequency, their transmission and absorption within certain media, and their effect on materials. Certain vibrations, whose amplitude is within known limits and whose frequencies fall within the range from about 20 to 16,000 Hertz (hz), can be perceived by the human ear and are, therefore, referred to as "sound."

According to this definition, the term *sound* refers only to vibrations of a certain frequency and amplitude and has a purely physiologic connotation.

Acoustic phenomena have measurable properties since mechanical vibrations have wave-like properties in regard to position, time, or both. A wave may be either simple or complex in form. Whatever the form of the wave, a mathematical technique called *Fourier analysis* can be employed to reduce it to the sum of sine and co-sine waves of appropriate amplitude and frequency.

The measurable properties are: (a) complexity of form; (b) amplitude; (c) wave length.

When acoustic waves travel in fluids, the energy of the wave is carried outwards by moving groups of molecules that have been alternately compressed and rarified by the vibrating source. A plot of the change in density of the fluid at a given point for a period of time would yield what we consider to be a *wave*. The velocity of propagation of the wave in a given fluid is approximately constant. The energy propagation of acoustic waves in fluids lends itself to the following detection scheme.

The moving mass of fluid exerts a pressure on a flat surface placed perpendicular to the direction of travel of the wave. The pressure varies directly with the density of the fluid striking the surface, and can be easily converted, first, to a *force,* and then to a *power* impinging on the flat surface. The pressure function can then be analyzed as it yields the measurable quantities previously discussed.

If we apply these techniques to sound, we should observe the following conditions:

1. The fluid should be air or, in special cases, water (blood);
2. Both the frequency and amplitude of the wave must fall within certain limits, which will be discussed below.

When we determine the range of frequencies that affect the auditory system of man, we find, for each frequency, upper and lower limits of amplitude beyond which the human ear does not yield the sensation of sound; there would be either no sensation (lower) or one described as pain (upper). These limits vary for each individual, and an idealized, average curve *(the auditory curve),* has been used as a standard. At each frequency of the auditory curve, the limits are so set that only a small percentage of the population would perceive as sound the waves that are outside these limits.

Within these limits, the following words have been used to qualitatively describe the sounds:

1. The *sound level* is proportional to the pressure or power density of the vibrations.
2. *Pitch* is a lay term related to the frequency of the vibrations.
3. The word *tone* describes the form of the wave.

While quantitation of sound level and pitch has been determined by experiment, tone does not lend itself to quantitation.

The analysis of *pitch* is accomplished in the following manner: A sound is generated which contains only one Fourier component, that is, a perfect sine wave or a "pure" tone. Pure tones are then generated at other frequencies which are a multiple of the original one. Subjects asked to describe a relationship between the tones generated in this way usually appreciate as an arithmetic progression (1,2,3,4,5, etc.) what was generated as a geometric progression (1,2,4,8,16, etc.) (Fig. 1). This means that the auditory system appreciates the change in frequency of a sound in a logarithmic fashion.

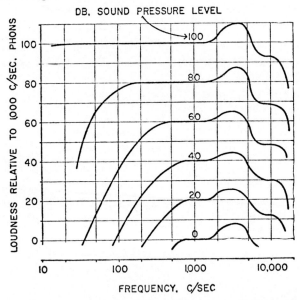

FIGURE 1. Loudness of several sound intensities at varying frequency. (From Fletcher—Speech and Hearing, Courtesy of the Van Nostrand Company of New York.)

The *fundamental frequency* is the lowest component frequency of a periodic quantity. It is equal to the inverse duration of the periodic pattern of a wave form.

A *harmonic* is a frequency component that is an integral multiple of the fundamental.

An *overtone* is a frequency component, higher than the fundamental, that is not an integral multiple of the latter.

The *intensity level of sound* was studied in a similar fashion.

However, the subjects report that one sound has *twice* the intensity level of another when the power density (or pressure) of the former is *ten times* that of the latter.

In a manner similar to pitch, the relationship between a pure tone of some power level and the same tone at power levels 10, 100, 1000, or 10,000 times greater have special significance. Indeed, if the intensity level of a pure tone is perceived as increased by equal steps, the power could be measured as increased by powers of 10 (Fig. 2). When we speak of sounds, rather than acoustic waves, we choose a conventional baseline of intensity level close to the lowest limits of hearing (10^{-16} watts/cm^2). The unit of intensity level is called *bel* and represents ten times the intensity level of the baseline. For example, a whisper in a quiet room is usually at an intensity level of 20 decibels (or 2 bels). In contrast, the rustle of leaves from trees is 10 decibels (or 1 bel). By comparison the following formulas are presented:

baseline intensity level $= 10^{-16}$ watts/cm^2

rustle of leaves $= 10^{-15}$ watts/cm^2

whisper $= 10^{-14}$ watts/cm^2

Therefore, for the rustle of leaves, the intensity in decibels equals

$$10 \log_{10} \frac{10^{-15}}{10^{-16}} \text{ or } 10 \log_{10} 10 \text{ or } 10\,(1) = 10$$

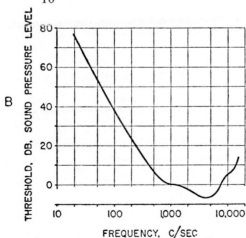

FIGURE 2. Variation of the threshold of hearing with frequency. Ordinate expressed in sound pressure level units, in which the reference is taken as 2×10^{-4} dynes/cm^2. (From Randall: *Elements of Biophysics,* courtesy of the Year Book Publ. Co., Inc. of Chicago.)

The range of intensity levels of sound includes over 12 orders of magnitude, that is, the most intense sound is more than 10^{12} times as intense as the least intense sound. As it is inconvenient to break up this huge span into just 12 steps, the decibel (or tenth of a bel) is used instead. The term decibel is usually abbreviated as *db*.

For acoustic waves in general, 10^{-16} has no specific importance, and *the sound intensity level in bels or decibels must be given relative to some stated value.*

One aspect of the *decibel scale* is that 3 db corresponds to a factor of 2 in power. That is, *if an acoustic wave is 3 db more intense than another, it contains twice the power; if it is 3 db less intense, it contains one-half of the power.* For this reason, most filters or amplifiers give data with respect to the 3 db point.

The *loudness* of a sound, that is, the intensity at which we

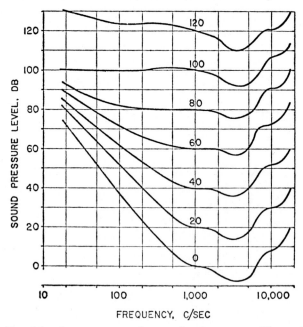

FIGURE 3. Equal loudness contours for varying frequency. The ordinate of a given curve is the intensity of a sound at each frequency, which must be presented to produce the sensation of loudness as a 1,000 Hz tone of the labeled pressure curve. (From Randall: *Elements of Biophysics,* courtesy of the Year Book Publ. Co., Inc. of Chicago.)

perceive sound, is not related in a simple fashion to the intensity level of the vibrations in decibels. The reason for this is that the human hearing apparatus does not respond in the same way to all frequencies. *A 1000 hertz pure tone at a level of 40 db would sound much louder to the average person than a 100 hertz pure tone at the same intensity level.* In other words, for sounds in the range of those created by the heart, an increase in frequency is usually perceived as an increase in loudness, even though the sounds have the same intensity level. For reasons such as this, a unit of loudness, *the phon,* has been created. This unit compares the loudness of a tone at a given frequency with the loudness of a tone at 1000 hz. The loudness of a given tone in phons is equal to the intensity level in decibels of a tone at 1000 hz that has the same apparent loudness (Fig. 3).

It has been observed that the heart sounds at the chest wall have a sound intensity level of more than 40 db. However, most of this sound phenomenon is produced at frequencies that are below 100 hz. Since the ear does not respond too well at 100 hz,

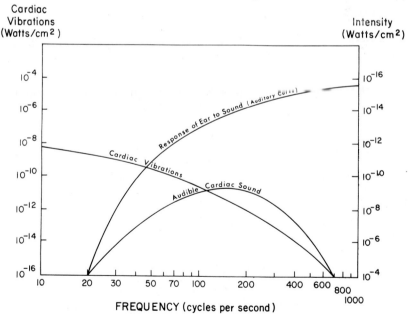

FIGURE 4. Average auditory curve compared with the average frequency of the cardiac sounds and resulting perception.

and the response is progressively worse below 100 hz, *the apparent loudness of the heart sounds is only about 5 phons,* i.e., *it has the same apparent loudness as a 1000 hz tone with an intensity level of only 4 db.*

It should be noted that sounds in a low band of frequencies (20 to 40 hz) may not be audible according to the threshold of hearing of the observer *(lower subliminal band).* On the other hand, murmurs in a high frequency band (500 to 1,500 hz) may or may not be audible according to the magnitude of the vibrations *(upper subliminal band).* The range between 40 and 500 hz is the one that includes most of the audible cardiac vibrations and is called, therefore, *auditory band* (Fig. 4).

Chapter 5

The Auditory System of Man

SOUND IS THE subjective interpretation of sensations produced by vibrations of air reaching the tympanic membrane
Chap. 4).

All statements about the auditory system are based on studies
involving large numbers of individuals. Although children may
detect sounds between 16,000 and 18,000 hz, adults seldom
detect them above 14,000 hz.

Auditory sensitivity is maximal between 1,000 and 2,000
hz, i.e., much above the usual range of cardiac sound. Below
1,000 hz, the sensitivity falls off rapidly, so that, to be heard, a
pure tone of 100 hz needs to have a sound pressure amplitude
about 100 times (40 db) greater than a pure tone of 1,000 hz.

The quality of sound is determined by four physical characteristics as follows:

1. *Pitch* relates to perception of changes in the frequency
   or number of vibrations per second.
2. *Intensity* relates to the magnitude of displacement of a
   sound wave; the more forceful the displacement, the
   greater the magnitude.
3. The presence and type of *harmonics* or *overtones* modifies the quality of sound.
4. *Duration* will determine whether a series of vibrations is

perceived as a "click" (or "snap"), a "tone," or a "murmur," the first being the shortest, the last being the longest.

Loudness is a purely physiologic aspect of sound because it is influenced by both frequency and magnitude.

The properties of the auditory system have been described by Fletcher and Munson, and the characteristics of the auditory system of man in regard to auscultation and phonocardiography have been investigated by Rappaport and Sprague, Butterworth *et al.,* and Ongley *et al.*

The sensitivity of the ear follows a non-linear curve so that *a sound having a higher pitch and the same intensity will be perceived as a louder sound until the frequency reaches about 1000 hz.*

Although the ear is able to function over an enormous range of pressure variations, it is a better detector of changes of pitch than of changes of intensity; however, in the lower frequency range, changes of pitch may not be detected at all.

In the presence of certain loud sounds, the ear is unable to detect other sounds that immediately follow. This phenomenon, called *masking* or *fatigue,* is revealed by recording sounds on tape and then playing the record in reverse; then a small sound, which normally follows a loud sound and is not heard, becomes audible (Butterworth *et al.*).

Binaural auscultation markedly increases the efficiency of perception. Other sensory stimuli (visual, etc.) should be avoided during auscultation because they may dull perception (in laymen's terms, they "distract the observer").

The importance of *decreasing ambient noise* as far as possible has been repeatedly emphasized because the *signal-to-noise ratio* (that will be discussed later in regard to phonocardiography) also applies to auscultation. It should be remembered that even a quiet room often has a noise level of 30 decibels, and a Hospital Ward up to 60 or 70 decibels.

Williams and Dodge reported detailed work on the frequency ranges of heart sounds, and Butterworth *et al.* made a detailed study of this problem.

The brain of a trained observer tends subconsciously to

select pertinent and meaningful information from the cardio-vascular point of view. Moreover, the brain is able to block out meaningless or undersized perception so that one can even listen to the heart sounds during respiration without being aware of the sounds related to the latter or even hear diastolic murmurs without hearing systolic murmurs. This selective process is well above the performance of a phonocardiograph because respiratory sound is still within the vibrational range of cardiac sound.*

A change of hearing is common with increasing age. It is customary to say that higher frequencies are less well perceived by older persons. This applies to frequencies encountered in music, however, and hardly ever to those generated by the heart. Therefore, persons who follow an ordinary conversation with difficulty are often well able to hear heart sounds and murmurs.

The *auditory appreciation of splitting* has been the object of investigation. The closest splitting that can be appreciated by the ear is that of two clicks made by the shutter of a camera at a 0.02 sec. or 20 msec. interval (Johnston). The magnitude and predominant frequency of the clicks found in practice, however, have great influence on the threshold. To be audible, the interval between the two components of the second sound is probably closer to 30 msec.

In conclusion, the auditory system of man is a marvelous apparatus which, however, is poorly suited for cardiac auscultation because of the characteristics of cardiac sound. In spite of this, training of the physician and conscious selection of certain phenomena considerably improve the results of auscultation and even (in particular cases) render it superior to phonocardiography. From all other points of view, phonocardiography is superior because its technical characteristics can be made to fulfill the job for which it has been developed.

---

*Modern technique would be able to include in an apparatus such a selective process in regard to periodic phenomena. This, however, would involve a great increase in price.

Our recent equipment has proven to be able to record heart sounds and murmurs during quiet respiration though not during noisy breathing.

Chapter 6

The Ear and the Stethoscope

THE EAR

IT IS SOMETIMES forgotten that the basic instrument of auscultation is the human ear.

The stethoscope was invented by Laennec for two primary reasons: (1) to avoid unpleasant contact with the unwashed skin of poor patients, and (2) to preserve the propriety of wealthy patients, particularly those of the female sex.

Even though the stethescope, particularly in its present form, has certain technical advantages, it often distorts, decreases, or selectively emphasizes certain vibrations. For these reasons, a good clinician should train himself to hear without the stethoscope, and should know the properties of the various stethoscopes.

The naked ear is often superior to the stethoscope in the detection of low-pitched vibrations (third sound, fourth sound) because of two properties: (1) the ear is a larger collector of sound; and (2) there is fusion of the auditory with the palpatory perception of the low-frequency vibrations.

THE STETHOSCOPE

Modern stethoscopes consist of: (1) the chest piece; (2) the tubing, and (3) the ear pieces.

Chest Piece

A chest piece may give different responses according to its

diameter, the ratio of diameter to height, and the presence or absence of a diaphragm.

The optimal diameter of a bell is about 2.5 cm for adults, 1.5 for children, and 1 cm for infants. The internal volume of air should be minimal, and therefore the depth of the bell should be as small as possible. A depth of 1.5 cm has been considered optimal (Rappaport and Sprague, Ongley *et al.*).

An *open bell* lightly applied on the skin is best suited for detecting low-pitched vibrations. Strong pressure of the bell would create a tense skin diaphragm that would filter out the low-pitched vibrations, thus giving emphasis to those of higher pitch. Actually, the latter seem louder only because they are not mixed with vibrations of a lower pitch (Rappaport and Sprague).

A *thin diaphragm* of 0.3 to 0.4 mm in thickness is excellent for the detection of high-pitched sounds and for appreciating split sounds and murmurs. It does so by acting as a *mechanical filter*. A thick membrane is the best for murmurs of the highest pitch but greatly attenuates their weak vibrations so that their auditory perception may be prevented.*

Tubing

The tubing should not be longer than 25 to 30 cm, and the total length of the stethoscope should not exceed 45 cm. Tubes with an internal bore of 3.0 to 3.2 mm seem to be the best (Rappaport and Sprague), and the material of the tubing should be semirigid to ensure that best conduction of sound.

Ear Pieces

Snug fitting of the ear pieces in the external auditory meatus of the observer's ears is essential. A slight change in the angle of application may reduce considerably the magnitude of the vibrations received by the tympanic membrane.

Binaural Stethoscope

The binaural stethoscope has several advantages over the old monaural type including a better fitting to the ears and a much greater efficiency. In the 60 to 700 hz range, binaural

---

*A similar membrane can be used with advantage in connection with microphones because increased amplification can compensate for this reduction.

audition is about 20 db (a tenfold increase) better than monaural (McKusick).

Historical developments of the stethoscope include the following:

1. The *rigid (wooden or metal) stethoscope* widely used in Europe even now (monaural) (Fig. 5A).

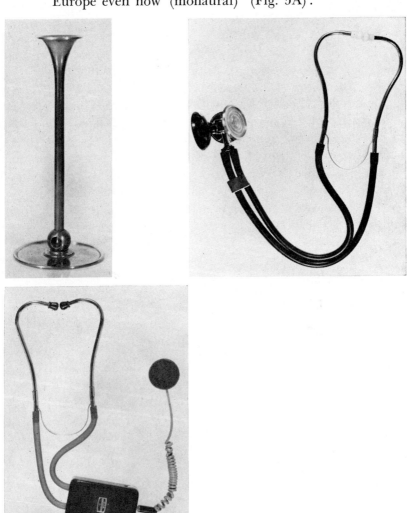

FIGURE 5. Stethoscopes. (a) Old monaural rigid stethoscope. (b) Modern stethoscope with three chest pieces. (c) Electronic stethoscope.

2. The *phonendoscope* of Bazzi-Bianchi (1898), a stethoscope with a chest piece closed by a diaphragm and binaural flexibile tubing.
3. The Bowles *diaphragm chest piece* (1901).
4. The *stethoscope* described by Sprague (1926) with both bell and diaphragm, which can be alternately used.
5. The *symballophone* of Kerr (1937) with two chest pieces; useful for comparison of sounds from two areas.
6. The *Sanborn stethoscope* with bell and diaphragm to be alternately used.
7. The *Tycos stethoscope* with three chest pieces (Fig. 5B).
8. The *Burch and Stock stethoscope,* especially designed for the high-frequency vibrations.

Amplifying Stethoscope

The amplifying (or electric) stethoscope is an electronic system similar to that employed in phonocardiography but used for either individual or collective auscultation. If it is provided with suitable microphone, filters, and amplifier, it may serve multiple purposes as follows:

1. Through amplification, it compensates for a defective auditory system.
2. Through amplification and selective filtration, it enables the observer to perceive either low-pitched sounds (lower subliminal band) or high-pitched sounds (upper subliminal band).
3. Through suitable amplification, it may partly overcome the phenomenon of masking.

It should be kept in mind that the amplifying stethoscope is not primarily intended for making sounds louder (though it may do so); rather it should be used to modify the inadequate characteristics of the auditory system through the judicious combination of amplification and selection.

Systems having these characteristics are available but are of large size and are unsuitable for clinical practice.* Smaller, pocket-size devices (Fig. 5C) are at present technically inadequate.

*A good apparatus is the portable Cambridge Audio-Visual Heart Sound Recorder, which also includes a small oscilloscope and a disk recorder.

NOISE LEVEL

Auscultation is deeply influenced by the noise level of the background.

According to Groom, the background noise of hospitals and clinics is rather constant, in the order of 60 to 70 decibels. Sounds and murmurs transmitted through ordinary stethoscopes are of relatively low intensity and are easily submerged or masked by extraneous noise. Simple sound-proofing measures may reduce the background noise by 50 per cent. Groom noted that a murmur that could be heard in a quiet room had to be increased more than 12 times to be detected under the average noise conditions of a hospital ward.

The signal-to-noise ratio will be discussed in Chapters 16 and 17.

The technique and art of auscultation have been re-emphasized by P. Harvey. The position of the physician, that of the patient, and an adequate system of examination are all important for extracting the essential data from this valuable method.

Part III

PHYSIOLOGY OF HEART SOUNDS AND MURMURS

Chapter 7

The Cardiac Cycle

A S ACTIVATION of the heart starts in the sinus node and procedes, first, to the atria, and then to the ventricles, it seems logical to describe the cycle in the same order (Figs. 4 and 6).

THE ATRIAL DYNAMICS

Atrial contraction occurs during the first 2/3 of the P-Q interval of the electrocardiogram at a time when about 5/6 of the diastolic filling has already occurred. It completes ventricular filling and causes a slight elevation of ventricular pressure.

Atrial relaxation starts during the latter portion of the P-Q interval. It is an important factor of atrioventricular valve closure because it permits the creation of a small ventriculo-atrial pressure gradient that is sufficient to approximate the floating leaflets of these valves. The pressure level existing in each ventricle at the end of the atrial cycle is called *end-diastolic pressure*, and corresponds to the *initial tension* of the ventricular muscle fibers.

VENTRICULAR CONTRACTION

At about the peak of the R wave of the electrocardiogram (or slightly before R), the ventricular septum, papillary muscles, and part of the ventricular walls are excited and start contracting.

A slow rise of pressure takes place in the ventricles during this initial period *(entrant phase* of Wiggers), and firm apposition of the AV valves leaflets takes place, aided by the increased chordal tension produced by contraction of the papillary muscles and of the intrinsic musculature of these leaflets, specially developed in the mitral valve.

The *isovolumic period* of ventricular contraction starts at this time. The entire musculature of the ventricles is contracting; the pressure rises rapidly because all valves are closed, and only a slight elevation of the valve structures and slight distension of the muscles of the ventricular base allows for acceleration changes of the blood contained in the cavities of the ventricles. The isovolumic period starts between R and S of the electrocardiogram and ends sometime after S, when the diastolic pressures of the pulmonary artery and of the aorta are reached, respectively. Brief oscillations of pressure are transmitted to the atria and to the large arteries by the closed valves during the isovolumic phase. As soon as the semilunar valves open, the *ejection phase* starts. Each ventricle forms like a single chamber with its main artery, and its pressure follows a rounded, flattish course. About 2/3 of ejection (or stroke volume) occurs during the first half of the phase. Subsequent to this, the rate of ejection decreases, and the pressure drops both in the large arteries and in the ventricles. The atrial pressures drop slightly during ventricular ejection, partly due to the suction created by the lowering of the atrio-ventricular floors, and partly to intrapericardial pressure changes induced by decreased ventricular volume.

VENTRICULAR RELAXATION

With cessation of ventricular contraction, the musculature of the ventricles relaxes rapidly. A slight backflow at the root of the large arteries causes the closure of the semilunar valves, and this is soon followed by a rebound of flow and pressure over the closed valves; this is evidenced by an *incisura* (drop in pressure) and a *secondary wave* (increase in pressure or *dicrotic wave*) in both the aorta and the pulmonary artery. There is a gross coincidence between the end of systole and the end of the T wave of the electrocardiogram.

THE INTERMEDIATE STAGE

The interval between the beginning of the incisura (end of

Figure 6. Scheme of the various phases of the cardiac cycle of man.

ECG = electrocardiogram

PCG = phonocardiogram

LV = left ventricle; RV = right ventricle; PA = pulmonary artery

LA = left atrium; RA = right atrium; Ao = aorta

I, II = first and second heart sound

III, IV = third and fourth heart sound

Mi, Tric = mitral and tricuspid valves

PA, Ao = pulmonary and aortic valves

Rt = right heart; Lt = left heart

(From Luisada and MacCanon, Amer. Heart J.)

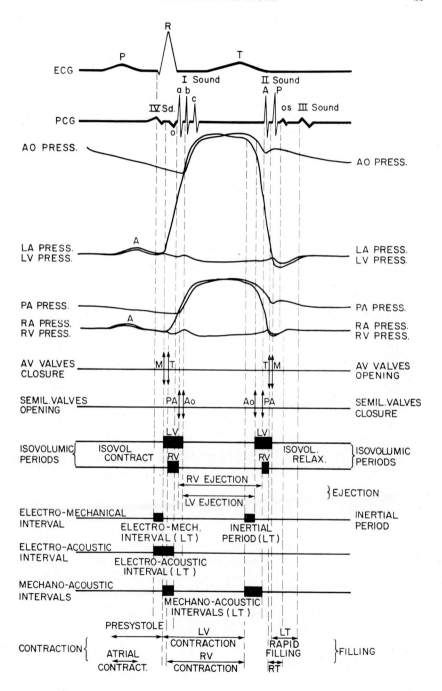

systole) and its trough has been called *protodiastole* by Wiggers. Following closure of the semilunar valves, the pressures drop rapidly in the ventricles until they fall below the levels of the atrial pressures. Then the atrioventricular valves open again. The interval between closure of the semilunar valves and opening of the AV valves is called *isovolumic relaxation period. Opening of the AV valves* is marked by a positive wave (*v* wave) in the atrial pressure curves. The *v* wave follows the closure of the semilunar valves and coincides with the beginning of diastole.

VENTRICULAR FILLING

As soon as the AV valves are open, a rapid drainage of atrial blood into the ventricles takes place. This may amount to ½ or more of the total filling. The first part of this *rapid filling* is aided by an active process, i.e., the release of elastic forces within the ventricular walls (Brecher). Filling then continues at a slower rate *(diastasis)* since distension of the ventricles causes tension of the papillary muscles and chordæ with narrowing of the AV valves.

At the end of diastasis, a new impulse starts at the SA node, and a new atrial contraction takes place completing ventricular filling.

ATRIOVENTRICULAR VALVE CLOSURE (Fig. 7)

The all important closure of the atrioventricular valves is obtained through several mechanisms.

1. Stretching of the papillary muscles and chordæ during diastasis narrows the opening of the tricuspid and mitral valves.
2. Eddies forming below the leaflets during the end of atrial contraction further narrow these valve openings.
3. Atrial relaxation permits the creation of a ventriculo-atrial gradient that closes the valves.
4. The early stage of ventricular contraction causes narrowing of the musculature around the valves; contraction of the intrinsic musculature of the valve leaflets renders them stiffer and more adherent to each other; and contraction of the papillary muscles induces tension of the chordæ that stiffens the entire valve apparatus.
5. Contraction of the ventricular septum and of the free wall

raises intraventricular pressure. This will tightly seal the valve leaflets, slightly push them toward the atria, and prevent any regurgitation. A slight upward rise of the valve rings and belly of the leaflets occurs but is soon checked by the downward pull of the chordæ.

DYNAMICS OF THE RIGHT AND LEFT HEARTS

The events of the two halves of the heart are not completely synchronous. Activation time for the two atria and ventricles is slightly different and the pressure levels of the ventricles and large vessels also differ. However, the delay between right and left atrial or ventricular events are very small (Tables III and IV).

CARDIOVASCULAR PRESSURES

The average pressures of the cardiac chambers and vessels have been studied by the author with Cortis in normal man and are reported in Table I.

TABLE I — AVERAGE PRESSURES (mm Hg)

Chamber or Vessel	RA	RV	PA	W	LA	LV	Ao
Pressures	3.2	20.9 / 2.5	19.0 / 6.7	8.26 (mean)	7.43 (mean)	103.9 / 6.7	106.9 / 68.4

RA = right atrium; RV = right ventricle
PA = main pulmonary artery; W = wedge pressure
LA = left atrium; LV = left ventricle; AO = aorta

ELECTROMECHANICAL INTERVALS

The electromechanical intervals were also measured and are reported in Table II.

TABLE II — AVERAGE ELECTRO-MECHANICAL INTERVALS
IN MILLISECONDS
(Corrected — 10 msec. were subtracted)

	QLV Rise	QAo Rise	QRV Rise	QPA Rise	QPA- QRV	QAo- QLV	QRV- QLV	QAo- QPA
Interval	30	68	47	61	14	38	17	7
Minimum	25	60	35	45	5	25	10	5
Maximum	35	70	55	70	15	35	20	10

DYNAMIC INTERVALS

On the basis of these measurements, the following dynamic intervals were obtained (Table III).

TABLE III — DYNAMIC INTERVALS IN MAN

Intervals in milliseconds between onset of QRS complex and onset of pressure rise after correction for catheter and electronic delay (10 msec. were subtracted)

$$QRV = 47$$

Isovolumic Period of Right Heart = 14

$$QPA = 61$$
$$QLV = 30$$

Isovolumic Period of Left Heart = 38

$$QAo = 68$$

Left ventricular-Right ventricular rise = 17

Sequence: LV — 30, RV — 47; PA — 67; Ao — 68.

TIMING OF VALVULAR EVENTS

The most likely timing of valvular events is listed in Table IV.

TABLE IV — PROBABLE AVERAGE TIMING OF VALVULAR EVENTS IN MAN IN MILLISECONDS AFTER CORRECTION FOR CATHETER DELAY (10 msec. were subtracted)

Interval Q-closure of Mitral valve	27
Interval Q-closure of Tricuspid valve	44
Interval Q-opening of Pulmonic valve	58
Interval Q-opening of Aortic valve	65

Chapter 8

Normal Heart Sounds and Their Mechanism

THE HEART sounds result from the interplay of the dynamic events associated with the heart beat and the blood flow.

During each phase of the cardiac cycle, the main directional mass movement of blood through the cavities of the heart and great vessels is determined and maintained as a function of the muscular and valvular apparatus. The interdependent work of the muscular and valvular systems is influenced to a great extent by the properties of the heart wall. The function of the hemodynamic system results in the generation of vibrations emanating from the pulsating heart and the pulsating vessels. The resultant energy produced is transmitted to the chest wall, where these vibrations are detected as heart sounds or murmurs.

The degree of audibility of these phenomena is largely dependent upon the quality of the interposed transmitting medium. Such vibrations are more attenuated in the regions insulated by a large compressible mass of lung tissue or in areas of the mediastinum containing accumulations of fat. They are more directly transmitted through relatively solid tissues or layers of minimal thickness, thus resulting in less attentuation of the heart sounds, which may consequently be picked up more readily.

Normal mammalians present *two* heart sounds by auscultation. Graphic tracings, however, may reveal up to *four* sounds and occasionally more, as illustrated in Figures 9, 10, 56-62. The

39

two louder sounds are called the first and second sounds; the two fainter, the third and fourth sounds.

The cardiac chambers and the large arterial vessels are filled with blood. As none of them can vibrate without producing movements or vibrations in the blood that they contain, the cardiac walls, valves, arterial walls, and blood represent an interdependent system that vibrates as a whole (Schuetz, Rushmer). Intracardiac phonocardiography (Luisada *et al.*, 1964, 1968; Guenther, 1969) shows that sounds created in one chamber are transmitted to the others with some loss of energy. This is particularly true of the large vibrations generated in the left heart, whereas the small vibrations theoretically created by the normal right heart at the beginning of systole are difficult or impossible to detect. In addition to being of minimal amplitude, they occur at the same time as the larger vibrations created by the left heart.

The concept of the mechanism of the heart sounds has greatly changed in the last 60 years. Originally noticed when the water pump with its simple valves represented the mechanistic model of the circulation, the theory that the heart sounds were caused by clapping of the valves at the time of their forceful closure is understandable. This theory was refused by Wiggers in 1915 when he lamented that "views propounded in Society Committees subsequently became so ingrained in the minds of physicians as to be extremely resistant to experimental or factual questioning." He stated the "the sudden elevation of intraventricular pressure produced by contraction sets many structures into vibration" and denied that "vibrations of different structures maintain their identity and can be identified in heart sound records."

A marked change in concept was proposed by Rushmer. According to him, the vibrations of the "cardiohemic system" are caused by acceleration and deceleration* of the blood (heart sounds). In an elastic chamber filled with fluid, any sudden motion throws the whole system into vibration. The momentum of the fluid would cause an overstretching of certain structures followed by a recoil and a displacement of fluid in the opposite

---

*The terms "acceleration" and "deceleration" should be viewed as meaning active forces which may be manifested as either pressure changes or actual physical displacement of blood or tissue.

direction. However, no experimental data were supplied at the time in support of this theory.

The intensity of a sound seems to be proportional to the rate of change of pressure, whereas the frequency of the sound seems to be connected with the relationship btween the size of the vibrating mass and the elasticity of the walls. In the heart, the combined mass (walls, blood, internal structures) is very large as compared to the elasticity.

Studies conducted in our laboratory have clarified the mechanism of the heart sounds and led to formulation of a theory that differs greatly from the old one. They have been subsequently confirmed or accepted by others including van Bogaert, Laurens, Dexter, B. Segal, Kingsley, and Guenther. They will be reported in detail in the following sections.

FIRST HEART SOUND

The mechanism of the production of the first heart sound has been repeatedly investigated. Many authors believed that the first heart sound was chiefly the result of a muscular vibration. Confirming previous studies, Wiggers and Dean, as well as Eckstein, recorded sound vibrations produced by the contraction of an isolated, perfused strip of myocardium. Kountz et al. (1940) eliminated valvular action by clamping the venæ cavæ wall for a few cycles and by blocking the atrioventricular orifices. A loud first sound was recorded until heart failure set in. However, the fact that most ventricular systole is unaccompanied by sound is against the theory of a muscular origin of the sound. The same type of experiment led others to believe that the first sound is purely the result of a valvular factor. Dock (1933) found that, following ligation of the atrioventricular groove or of the venæ cavæ and the azygos, there was either disappearance or extreme reduction of the first sound. He concluded that the latter is caused by "the sudden tension of the previously slack fibers of the A-V valves." Smith et al. (1950), on the basis of experiments on surviving perfused dog hearts, reached the conclusion that the first sound is largely due "to the forceful striking of the valves." It should be noted that the two above views are incompatible because valve closure precedes in time valve tension. Moreover, valve closure occurs gently and gradually while valve tension is more sudden and abrupt.

Orías and Braun-Menendez stated that the first sound consisted of separate vibrations caused by atrial, valvular, muscular, and vascular factors, and Rappaport and Sprague (1942) agreed with this concept.

A study of the mechanism of production of the first sound was made by Luisada *et al.* (1952) in open-chest experiments. Several types of experiments were performed on the empty heart after ligation of the atrioventricular groove, severe damage to one or both atrioventricular valves, ligation of the large arterial vessels, or myocardial necrosis. It was concluded that "extensive damage of either the A-V valves or the ventricular walls caused extreme reduction in the intensity of the first heart sound."

Emphasis on valvular factors is found in the studies of Leatham and Towers and of Leatham (1954). It is known that the first sound of normal subjects or cardiac patients may be audibly split. Leatham attributed the normal close splitting of the first sound to the sequence of a "mitral" and a "tricuspid" component. He also described a high-pitched vibration in early systole of clinical cases, which he named "ejection click" (aortic or pulmonary according to the underlying disease). While Leatham at first considered "valve closure" as the cause of the first heart sound, later he accepted "valve tension" as the basic factor.

It is interesting to note that, while many clinical cardiologists of the last twenty years were moving closer to a valvular theory, several physiologists were moving in the opposite direction.

The first heart sound is initiated by a few low-frequency vibrations and is terminated by a variable number of low-frequency vibrations in decrescendo. The beginning of the first sound is marked by a small, slow deflection that we call *o* (Figs. 9, 10). This component is probably caused by changes in the form of the ventricular mass *(entrant phase)*. The terminal vibrations of the first sound are explained by vibrations of the walls of the great vessels during the first part of ejection. This led us (Luisada *et al.*, 1949) to suggest division of the first sound into three sections, the central being of greatest interest for auscultatory correlations. This central part is formed by both medium- and high-frequency vibrations while the first and the last are formed by vibrations of a low frequency.

Experiments in our laboratory have cast new light on the mechanism of the first sound. Studies of Di Bartolo *et al.* (1961)

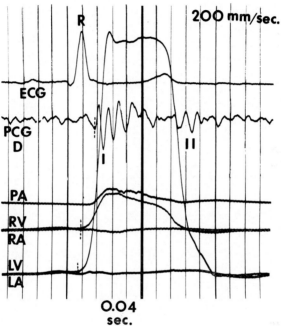

FIGURE 7. Valve closures, pressures, and sounds. Experiment in a dog with pressure tip sensors. RV-RA crossing = closure of tricuspid value. LV-LA crossing = closure of mitral valve. Displacement phonocardiogram (Pcg-D) showing the sharp largest early vibration of the first heart sound.

demonstrated that both the mitral and the tricuspid valves are already closed at the time of the first rapid vibration of the first sound* (Fig. 7). Subsequent experiments were performed in

---

*The closure of the AV valves seems to be caused largely by an atrial mechanism if there is a sinus rhythm, as proved by Sarnoff *et al.* In cases of atrial fibrillation or AV block, closure of the AV valves is completed by the rise of ventricular pressure as a result of the early phase of ventricular systole. Even here, however, there is a delay between closure of the valves and most of the rapid rise of pressure.

Mitral valve closure (revealed by crossing of the left atrial and left ventricular pressure curves) is completed during the Q-R ascending branch. The first slow group of vibrations of the first sound (component *o*) occurs about 10 msec. later during the first part of the R-S descending branch. The first group of large and rapid vibrations of the first heart sound (component *a*) occurs about 20 to 25 msec. after mitral valve closure in the dog, about 30 to 35 msec. in man. This interval was confirmed through angiocardiographic studies by Criley *et al.* (1962a) and also by MacCanon *et al.* (1969).

animals with functional exclusion of one ventricle. Exclusion of the right ventricle (Luisada *et al.* 1967) was *not* followed by modification of the first heart sound of the left ventricle (Fig. 11). Exclusion of the *left* ventricle was followed by *complete disappearance of the first heart sound* of the right ventricle even though this ventricle was strongly contracting (Luisada *et al.,* 1968) (Fig. 12). As a result of these studies, the first component of the normal first sound was explained as coinciding with the rapid rise of pressure within the left ventricle, which causes sud-

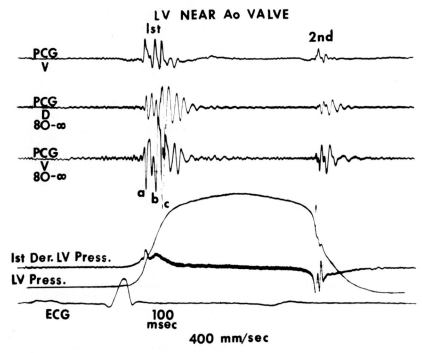

FIGURE 8. Relationship between heart sounds and pressure tracings. Experiment in a dog with pressure tip catheter either in the outflow tract of the left ventricle just below the aortic valve (A) or just above the aortic valve (B). *From above:* Unfiltered external phonocardiogram (apex); fiiltered phonocardiogram (apex), displacement (slope 48 db/octave); filtered phonocardiogram (apex), velocity (slope 48 db/octave); pressure; first derivative of pressure; electrocardiogram. Filtered tracings are delayed 12 msec.; unfiltered tracing, 4 msec.; pressure tracing, 4 msec. The second component of the first sound coincides with the onset of pressure rise in the root of the aorta.

den tension of the ventricular walls, septum, chordæ, and closed mitral valve. The explanation of the other components of the first sound was suggested by other experiments in dogs (Shah *et al.*, 1963), which showed coincidence of the various components with changes in rapidity of the left ventricular pressure curve. Experiments of MacCanon *et al.* (1969) with high speed cineangiocardiography and phonocardiography have confirmed the existence of a sizable interval between actual "closure" of the mitral valve and first heart sound. They also have permitted

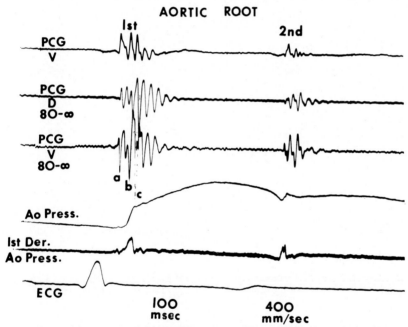

to evaluate the part played by "tension" of the mitral valve in the energy content of the first heart sound. Correlation of the valve surface, valve mass and excursion, and energy of the first sound revealed that the valve (including chordæ and papillary muscles) contributes only about 10 per cent of the total energy (Fig. 13).

Most of the vibrations of the heart sounds are caused by acceleration phenomena, a theory first advanced by Rushmer.

As the terms "acceleration" and "deceleration" are used to explain the various sounds originating in the cardiovascular system, it becomes necessary to define these terms more precisely than has usually been done until now.

One of the most common measurements that is made in the study of the heart and great vessels is the pressure in these structures. A *pressure* measurement is a measurement of force per

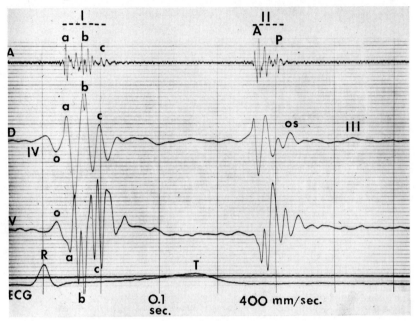

FIGURE 9. Phonocardiograms of a normal young man recorded with calibrated equipment recording tracings of displacement (D), velocity (V), and acceleration (A). a,b,c—the three main high frequency components of the first sound. A,P—the two main high frequency components of the second sound. O—low frequency component initiating the first sound. OS = slow vibration coincident with opening of mitral valve. III, IV = third and fourth sounds.

unit area, so that we are essentially measuring *force*. This force is ultimately traceable to the muscles of the heart which contract and relax to pump the blood. The force is chiefly exerted on the blood of the left ventricle. When this blood leaves the ventricle, it in turn exerts a force on the arterial system. When the blood leaves the ventricle through the aortic valve, it goes from a motionless state within the ventricle to a state of motion in the aorta. This change of velocity is called *acceleration*. When the blood enters the aorta, it slows down, and thus suffers a *negative*

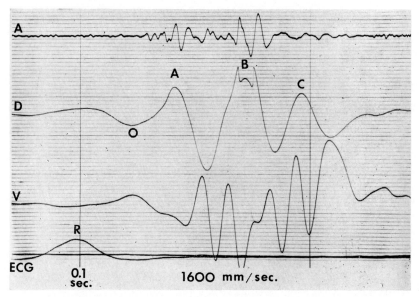

FIGURE 10. (a) First heart sound. (b) Second heart sound. The tracings are phonocardiograms of acceleration (A), displacement (D), and velocity (V) at a film speed of 1600 mm/sec.

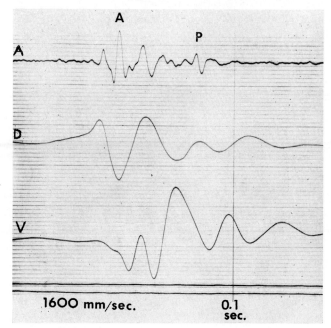

acceleration or "deceleration." When the left ventricle contracts, a force is exerted on the blood it contains causing an acceleration of the blood and a simultaneous deceleration (negative acceleration) of the heart muscle.

After opening of the aortic valve, the pressure in the aorta increases as the blood enters it, and then decreases. When the arterial pressure increases, the walls of the system experience an outward acceleration. When the pressure falls, the walls of the system experience an inward acceleration, caused by their own elastic and muscular reaction. Whenever there is a "deceleration" of the blood this is accompanied by an "acceleration" of the walls.

The important factors which concern the sounds of the heart are those which change the energy state of the walls of the system, since it is from the walls that all the energy is transduced.

So, the acceleration or deceleration of the blood, walls, valves, or any other structure must be considered in the context of the vibrations and resonances of the walls of the system.

The beginning of the first heart sound is revealed by a small low-frequency vibration *(component o),* which occurs at about the R wave of the electrocardiogram and at or slightly before the onset of rise of left ventricular pressure. Following this, there is the most important phase, that of the high frequency vibrations, which is the central phase of the first heart sound.

This central phase of the first heart sound contains three groups of rapid vibrations or components.

1. A rapid, early *first component* occurs between R and S of the electrocardiogram and follows the closure of the mitral valve by about 30-40 msec. in man. It coincides with the first part of the rapid rise in pressure recorded within the left ventricle. It is *called component a* (Fig. 7).

2. A *second rapid component* occurs 25 to 40 msec. later and coincides with a change in rate of the rise of pressure as revealed by the first derivative of the latter. It coincides with the opening of the aortic valve and is *called component b* (Fig. 8b).

3. A *third component* is often present about 60-70 msec. after the first. It coincides with a peak of pressure within the ascending aorta and is maximal above the aortic valve, even though it is well recorded also in the outflow tract of the left ventricle.

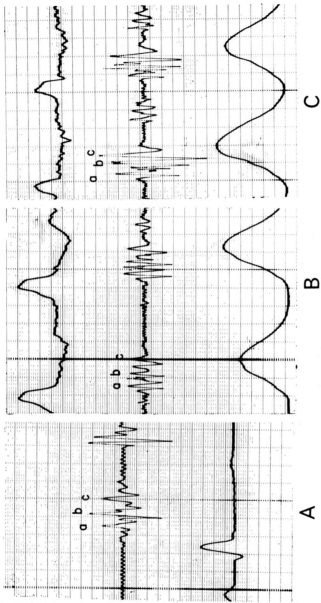

FIGURE 11. Experiment in a dog with right heart bypass. (A) Heart sounds recorded at the apex before opening the chest. Three components of the first heart sound (a,b, and c) are present (upper tracing). External phonocardiogram (lower tracing). Electrocardiogram. (B and C) Heart sounds recorded from within the left ventricle during the bypass. Three components of the first heart sound (a,b, and c) are still recorded. Tracings from above down are electrocardiogram, left ventricular intracardiac phonocardiogram, and left ventricular pressure tracing. Time lines = 40 msec.; recorded at 200 mm/sec. (From Luisada et al.: Circulation, 1967, courtesy of the Amer, Heart Assoc.)

It is *called component c* (Fig. 8b).

4. With microphones recording low frequency vibrations, a *fourth component,* called *d,* that coincides with the peak of expansion of the aorta, is recorded (Fig. 60).

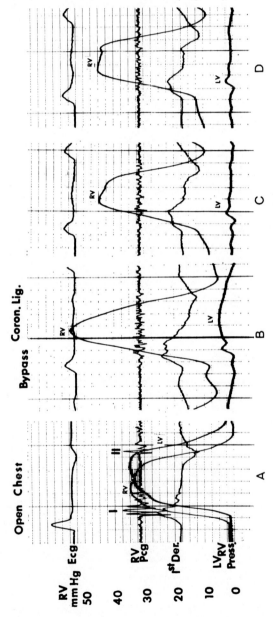

The first high frequency component (a) is of left ventricular origin and occurs during the first part of the isovolumic tension period (Fig. 17). The magnitude of this component has been correlated with the level of left ventricular pressure rise and with the rapidity of this rise (dp/dt) (Figs. 14-16).

The second high frequency component (b) also occurs within the left ventricle. The most plausible explanation is that it is caused by the sudden decrease in tension of the ventricular wall and the sudden increase in acceleration of the blood when the mitral valve opens (Fig. 8b).

The third component (c) occurs when there is a sudden change in the slope of the aortic pulse related to acceleration of aortic flow (Fig. 8b).

The fourth component (d) occurs during the maximal distension of the aortic wall (Fig. 60) and is only occasionally found.

While the first two components are caused by vibrations of the left ventricular wall, septum, papillary muscles, chordæ, and the closed tensing mitral valve plus their left ventricular blood, the last two are mainly caused by vibrations of the aorta with its blood.

A *close splitting* of the first sound (components a and b) is a normal phenomenon, both on auscultation and in phonocardiographic tracings. The interval between a and b is not modified

---

FIGURE 12. Records from an experimental dog. (A) Right ventricular pressure and phonocardiogram are recorded with a Dallons-Telco micromanometer placed in the center of the right ventricle. The first derivative of the right ventricular pressure is obtained through an analog computer circuit. Left pressure is recorded by means of a catheter introduced in the left ventricle through an apical puncture and a Statham strain gauge. Amplification of left ventricular pressure is $\frac{1}{4}$ of that of the right ventricle (the apparent delay between the two pressure curves is due to catheter delay in the case of the left ventricle). (B) Records obtained after left heart bypass and ligature of the circumflex branch of left coronary artery. Marked reduction in the amplitude of the heart sounds of the right ventricle. (C) Records obtained after withdrawing of residual blood from the left ventricle. (D) Records obtained after opening the cavity of the left ventricle. Complete disappearance of the heart sounds of the right ventricle. (From Luisada et al.: J. Appl. Physiol., 1968, courtesy of the Publisher.)

by respiration (Sainani *et al.* 1969) confirming that the two components originate in the same ventricle, the left. A *wide splitting* (components *a* and *c*, b absent) of the first sound is abnormal on auscultation but is not uncommon in the phonocardiogram, especially if the subject is a mature or elderly person (Fig. 18).

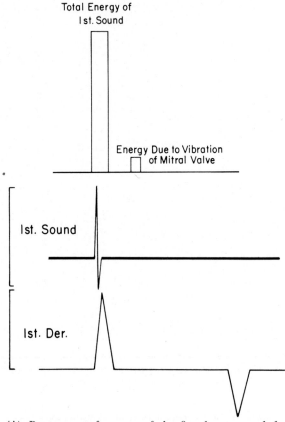

FIGURE 13. (A) Percentage of energy of the first heart sound due to tension of the mitral valve. (B) Relationship of the main high frequency component of the first heart sound with the first derivative (dp/dt) of the left ventricular pressure curve.

In a study conducted with a new calibrated system, Sakai *et al.* have found a marked variability in the amplitude of the a and b components of the first sound at various frequencies in different normal subjects. However, the maximum amplitude was usually found between 20 and 40 Hz.

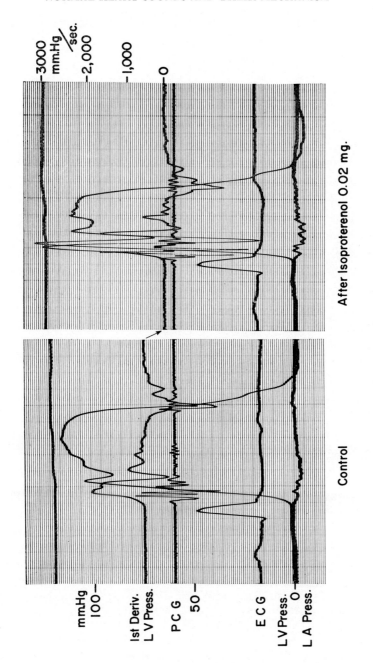

FIRST HEART SOUND AND CARDIAC FUNCTION

Physically, sound is produced by a force which throws structures into vibration. Whatever the origin, the heart sounds must arise from forces generated within the heart, the great vessels, or both. The left ventricular pressure rise may be regarded as a manifestation of contractile force which, except for the resistance offered, would have accelerated the blood into the aorta. Prevented from doing this by the closed valves, the left intraventricular blood mass is rapidly decelerated. Thus, the contractile energy tending to accelerate the blood is converted into the potential energy of pressure during isovolumic contraction. As tension or stretch has been shown to induce sonic vibrations, it seems reasonable to relate the first heart sound to these events. As mitral tension and excursion alone cannot account for the sonic energy, and since the left ventricular wall oscillates in phase with the first sound, the left ventricle (walls, boundaries, and content) can be considered as a unit transducer analogous to the cone of a loudspeaker.

The percentage change in the magnitude of the first component of the first sound has been correlated with the level of left ventricular pressure and with the percentage change in the amplitude of the first systolic wave of the first derivative of left ventricular pressure. A linear correlation was found between the first component and the first derivative of LV pressure suggesting a strong relationship between the first sound and the rapidity of left ventricular contraction (Sakamoto *et al.,* 1965) (Figs. 14-16).

A study of the first sound in patients with a prosthetic Starr valve replacing the mitral valve has been made by Shah *et al.* (1963a). High-speed recording of the closure sound of such a

---

Figure 14. Typical effect of *isoproterenol* showing proportional increases of the first sound and of the first derivative (dp/dt) of the left ventricular pressure in the absence of large change in systolic pressure. *From above:* Respiratory tracing (not labelled), first derivative of left ventricular pressure (1st Deriv. L.V. Press.), external phonocardiogram (P.C.G.), electrocardiogram (E.C.G.), left ventricular pressure (L.V. Press.), and left atrial pressure (L.A. Press.). Pressure scale (mm Hg) is on the left. Pressure derivative scale (mm Hg/sec.) is on the right. (From Sakamoto *et al.:* Circulation Res. 1965, courtesy of the Amer. Heart Assoc.)

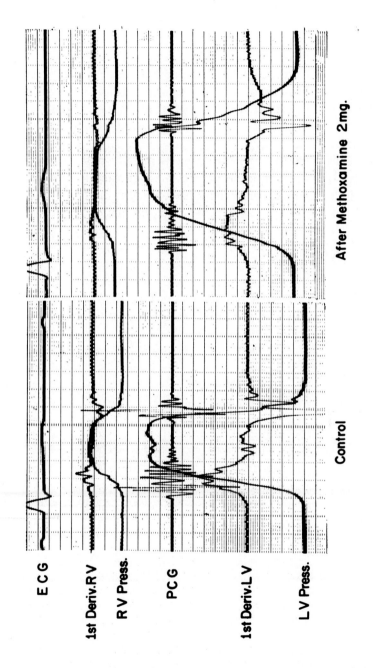

ECG

1st Deriv. RV

RV Press.

PCG

1st Deriv. LV

LV Press.

Control

After Methoxamine 2mg.

valve showed that this vibration arrived first in the third or fourth left interspace close to the sternal border and later at the apex. The area of first arrival coincided with the projection of the prosthetic valve on the chest wall as indicated by x-ray. However, the first component of the first heart sound is known to arrive earlier at the apex (Faber and Burton). This indicates that the first component of the normal first sound has a source other than the mitral valve.

Many studies have indicated that only a small fraction of the information available at the chest surface is currently utilized to evaluate cardiac action. These evaluations are mostly based on empirical impressions and pattern recognition, which only allow qualified estimates of heart dynamics. Investigations in this laboratory in 1965 (Sakamoto *et al.*) demonstrated that experimentally-induced changes (drugs, surgery, etc.) in the amplitude of the first heart sound are closely correlated with changes in the systolic peak of the first derivative (dp/dt) or left ventricular pressure rise (Figs. 14-16). Other workers (Reeves *et al.*, Gleason and Braunwald) have related this maximal rate of left ventricular pressure rise to cardiac contractility. These findings suggest that first heart sound recorded in calibrated absolute value terms would provide a useful means of assessing the status of cardiac function. However, many of the biophysical factors involved in the production of the first heart sound and in the transmission of these vibrations to the chest surface still need to be clarified.

The long-term goal of the phonocardiographic studies is to develop a reliable method of determining the losses involved in the transmission of heart sounds to the chest surface and to clarify the relationship between the first heart sound, the size of

---

FIGURE 15. Typical effect of *methoxamine* showing a proportional decrease in amplitude of the first heart sound and of the first derivative (dp/dt) of left ventricular pressure although arterial pressure is increased. *From above:* Electrocardiogram (E.C.G.), first derivative of right ventricular pressure (1st Deriv. R.V.), right ventricular pressure (R.V. Press.), external phonocardiogram (P.C.G.), first derivative of left ventricular pressure (1st Deriv. L.V. Press.), and left ventricular pressure (L.V. Press.). (From Sakamota *et al.*: Circulation Res., 1965, courtesy of the Amer. Heart Assoc.)

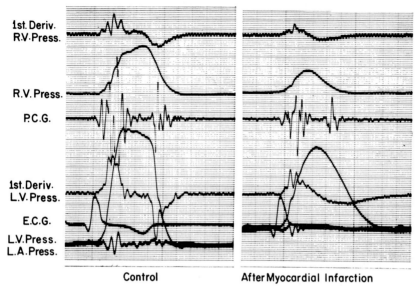

1st. Deriv.
R.V. Press.

R.V. Press.

P.C.G.

1st. Deriv.
L.V. Press.

E.C.G.

L.V. Press.
L.A. Press.

Control   **After Myocardial Infarction**

FIGURE 16. Typical effect of *myocardial infarct* (embolization of the coronary arteries with plastic microspheres) showing proportional reduction in amplitude of the first heart sound and of the first derivative (dp/dt) of left ventricular pressure while systolic pressure is reduced. *From above:* First derivative of right ventricular pressure (1st Deriv. R.V. Press.), right ventricular pressure (R.V. Press.), external phonocardiogram (P.C.G.), first derivative of left ventricular pressure (1st Deriv. L.V. Press.), electrocardiogram (E.C.G.), left ventricular pressure (L.V. Press.), and left atrial pressure (L.A. Press.). (From Sakamota *et al.*: Circulation Res., 1965, courtesy of the Amer. Heart Assoc.)

the heart, and the energetics of cardiac contraction. Measurements of the phase relations of pressure and sound events in various portions of the left ventricle using miniature transducers confirmed Faber's impression that the ventricular walls vibrate in phase with the blood. However, more refined experiments are in progress to distinguish wall acceleration from blood deceleration. Other experiments indicate a decrease in first heart sound frequency and mplitude as heart size increases as long as peak dp/dt of left ventricular pressure does not change.

As encouraging as these results have been, the need to develop better transducing and recording equipment and automated anlaytical method for handling the complexities of the problem

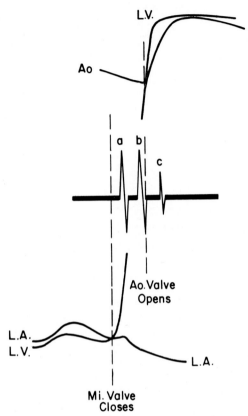

FIGURE 17. Time relationship between the three components of the first heart sound and the dynamic events of the left heart and aorta (scheme).

became obvious in 1968. This problem was solved in collaboration with the Research and Development Section of the General Electric Company of Schenectady, New York, which led to development and construction of a new apparatus.

Studies in dogs have been undertaken with this system. Heart sounds have been measured at the chest surface, muscle, pleura, lung, pericardium and surface. The purpose of these measurements is to determine the transmission characteristics of these structures, and thus learn more of the mode of tissue "transduction" and correlate surface energy with that produced at the heart (Chap. 10).

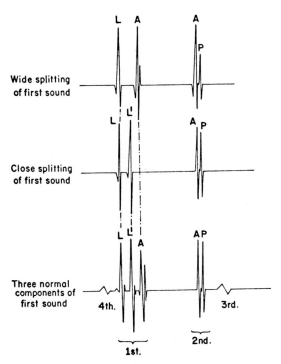

FIGURE 18. Two different types of splitting of the first heart sound. Wide splitting is caused by audition of the first (a or L) and third (c or A) while close splitting is caused by audition of the first and second (a and b, or L and L').

THE ABNORMAL FIRST HEART SOUND

The first heart sound may *decrease* in amplitude if: (1) the left ventricle is weak; (2) the left ventricle is markedly enlarged; (3) part of its energy is absorbed by elastic structures, or (4) its pressure rise is slower for hemodynamic reasons.

Weakness of the left ventricle is found in left heart failure, where the rise of pressure is slower and may reach a lower peak. If the ventricle is markedly dilated on account of failure, there will be three causes for decrease of the first sound (lower peak, slower rise, and larger ventricle). Marked dilatation also occurs in severe aortic or mitral insufficiency. As, in mitral insufficiency, the leak through the mitral valve decreases the rapidity of pressure rise, two different causes (large left ventricle, slower rise

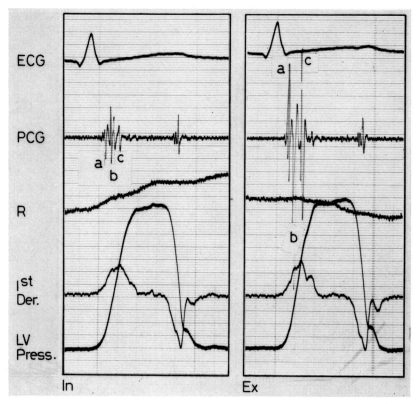

FIGURE 19. Changes of the first heart sound in inspiration (In) and expiration (Ex) in a dog. The first derivative shows several notchings coinciding with the three components of the first heart sound.

because of leak) will be present. However, ventricular hypertrophy may compensate and even overcompensate for these factors so that the first sound in mitral insufficiency may be normal or even increased. In aortic insufficiency, ventricular dilatation tends to decrease the first sound but compensatory hypertrophy may reestablish the normal amplitude. Following a myocardial infarct, part of the energy of contraction of the left ventricle is absorbed by the necrotic or scarred tissue. This will decrease the rapidity of pressure rise and thus the amplitude of the first sound. For this reason, a softer first sound in myocardial infarct does not necessarily define left ventricular failure. On the other hand, such weakness is often present and is a concurrent cause of decrease of the first heart sound.

The first heart sound may *increase* in amplitude if: (1) there is greater resistance to stretch of certain structures (less compliance, greater rigidity) ; (2) the left ventricle is small; (3) the left ventricle is hypertrophied, or (4) there is an increased rapidity of contraction. Greater resistance to stretch is found in mitral stenosis where the mitral ring and the mitral valve are fibrosed or calcified. This will cause a more rapid rise of pressure during the tension period but only after the left atrial pressure level has been reached (late and louder first sound). A small left ventricle would cause vibrations of a higher frequency and greater amplitude. This will be a second cause for a larger and louder first sound in mitral stenosis, particularly because vibrations of higher frequency are perceived by the ear as "louder" vibrations. Ventricular hypertrophy tends to cause larger sound. This will occur in systemic hypertension, coarctation, aortic stenosis, or aortic insufficiency unless other factors (failure, fibrosis, valve leaks) tend to cause the opposite effect. Increased rapidity of contraction may be caused by hyperthyroidism, stimulation of the sympathetic system, or drugs which stimulate the myocardium or cause either a direct or a reflex sympathetic stimulation (isoproterenol, epinephrine, amyl nitrite) .

A *varying amplitude* of the first heart sound is found in atrial fibrillation, A-V block, and ectopic beats. It can be explained by the combination of various factors: the left ventricle has a different size for each beat on account of different previous filling; it exerts a different force of contraction, largely related to different filling; and has a longer or shorter isovolumic period according to the level of aortic pressure it has to overcome. In addition, ventricular pressure rise will find the mitral valve in different positions and will be the main factor of valve closure. As a result, functional mitral insufficiency is often present and the rapidity of pressure rise will greatly vary. Thus a multiplicity of factors will play a role in causing changes of the first heart sound in arrhythmias and blocks.

SECOND HEART SOUND

The closure of the semilunar valves was suggested as the

essential cause of the second heart sound by Rouanet (1832).
Wiggers (1915) believed in a silent closure of the semilunar
valves followed by the second sound. Leatham and Towers, and
Leatham (1954), by simultaneous recordings from various
auscultatory areas of the precordium, concluded that closure of
the aortic and pulmonary valves is responsible for the two main
components of the second sound (wherever they are heard or
recorded), and that splitting of the sound is caused by asynchro-
nous closure of these valves.

Although the valvular origin of the second sound has been
generally accepted in recent years, positive experimental evidence
is scarce and the actual mechanism involved still needs to be
clarified. Experiments with epicardial phonocardiography have
shown that the pulmonary artery receives and transmits well the
aortic component of the second sound. Clinical intracardiac
phonocardiograms frequently show *both components of the second sound in the right ventricle and atrium and in the pulmonary artery* (Luisada *et al.*, 1964; Guenther, 1969). These
studies indicate that the aortic component of the second sound is
frequently transmitted to the right heart, whereas the reverse
is less common.

In an experimental study of our laboratory (Mori *et al.*), the
problem has been investigated by means of intracardiac phonocardiograms (phonocatheters introduced into the aortic root and
pulmonary artery near the valves) plus pressure tracings, external phonocardiograms, and electrocardiograms. Both in the aorta
and the pulmonary artery there can be one, two, or three components of the second sound. When one component is present,
it is closely associated with the incisura of the pressure pulse of
the vessel in which it is recorded. When two components are
present, they coincide with the two incisuras and should be
labeled as *A (aortic)* and *P (pulmonic)* according to the vessel of
origin. The A component originates in the aorta and is well transmitted to the pulmonary artery whereas the P component originates in the pulmonary artery and is poorly transmitted to the
aorta because of its smaller magnitude and the thicker wall of
the aorta. In the aorta of some animals, there is also an X *component* preceding the aortic component by an average of 7 msec.

(Fig. 20). A small X component can be found occasionally in the external phonocardiogram and also within the left ventricle of animals and man. It may be explained by a vibration of the left

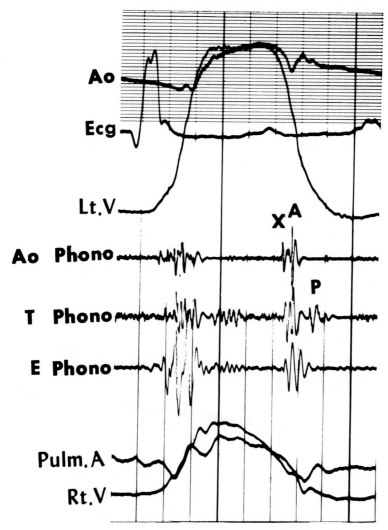

FIGURE 20. Tracings of intracardiac pressures and heart sounds in a normal dog. The three phonocardiograms from above are intravascular aortic, intratracheal, and external. The P component is visible in the tracheal tracing. The X component and the A component are visible in the aortic tracing.

(From Mori *et al.:* Cardiologia, 1964, courtesy of the Publisher.)

ventricular wall when the systolic contraction ceases and the pressure drops rapidly.

In studies on ventricular ejection, Spencer and Greiss showed that, at the moment in which blood flow reverses its course in the ascending aorta, the aortic pressure pulse begins the sharp drop that ends in the incisura, so that a sharp wave of backflow corresponds to this notch or trough. At this moment, abrupt cessation of the backflow occurs, and the aortic pressure rises to a sharp peak as a rebound wave. It is logical to assume that the aortic valve starts to close at the moment in which the blood flow reverses its course and that closure is well completed by the time of the incisura. A study of MacCanon *et al.* has shown that closure of the aortic valve occurs about 9 msec. *before* the aortic incisura, whereas the study of Mori *et al.* has revealed that the A component is very near the incisura. Thus, the sound phenomenon occurs *after* the closure of the aortic valve.*

Faber and Purvis concluded that the aortic component of the second heart sound originates and is transmitted as a transverse vibration of the aortic wall, which is inseparable from the high-frequency components of the aortic incisura. It seems that the abrupt cessation of backflow occurring at the time of the incisura sets into vibration the blood column, the valve, the arterial wall, and the infundibulum of the left ventricle (cardiohemic system) producing the sound.

Okino and Spencer (personal communication) obtained similar findings in regard to the dynamics of both the aortic and the pulmonary valves. A sequence of events, similar to that admitted for the A component, should then be considered in the production of the P component.

The main difference between aortic and pulmonary components is that the incisura of the pulmonary artery is caused by an elastic reaction that is much weaker (low pressure-high velocity). Therefore, a longer interval between pulmonary valve closure and pulmonic component of the second sound is usually found.

Normal inspiration does not appreciably change the dura-

---

*Studies of van Bogaert led him to a different conclusion. However, his observations can be criticized on technical grounds and do not alter the above interpretation.

tion of right ventricular systole. However, greater distension of the pulmonary artery, caused by larger blood flow, causes a delay in the rebound and thus a delay in the timing of the pulmonary component.

In 1949, the author with Mendoza suggested division of the second heart sound into three phases:

(a) An *early phase,* which has vibrations of a lower frequency; the component X can be recorded in this phase;

(b) A *central phase,* which is made of high frequency vibrations and contains the vibrations of the components A (aortic) and P (pulmonic);

(c) A *final phase,* which is again made of low frequency vibrations; this occasionally contains a larger vibration that closely follows in time the opening of the mitral valve; the author has considered this as the physiologic counterpart of the opening snap and has called it *opening sound* (OS) (Fig. 21).

Studies of Kusukawa *et al.* in our laboratory have indicated that the intensity of the second sound is related to the inertial energy involved in the deceleration of backflow. This, in turn, is determined by vessel wall elasticity, systolic runoff of the preceding stroke volume, and the rapidity of ventricular relaxation. Evidence for this was obtained in experimental animals subjected to various procedures or injected with drugs in order to alter cardiovascular dynamics. These studies showed that the intensity of the aortic component of the second sound is linearly related to the rate of development (first derivative) of aortic-to-left-ventricular differential pressure rather than to the arterial pressure level per se.

According to a number of studies and our own observations, *duration of the Q-II interval (Q-IIA or Q-IIP, respectively) is prolonged by either diastolic or systolic overload of a ventricle.* Any, even minor, degree of failure would further increase this duration. The increase in the duration of Q-II is far greater in clinical cases, where the process has lasted for a long time, than in acute animal experiments. The effect is again greater for the right heart than for the left because RV diastolic overload, through distension of the weak-walled pulmonary artery, causes a much greater delay in the occurrence of the P component.

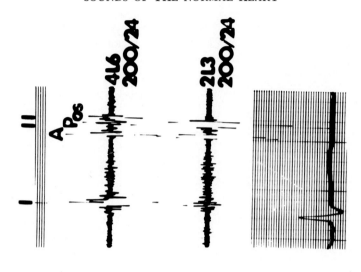

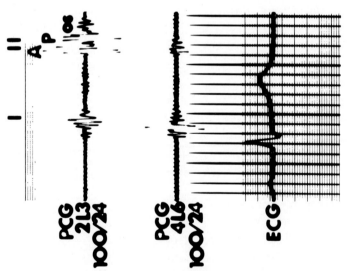

FIGURE 21. Physiologic opening sound of mitral valve in two young people (17 and 11 years respectively) with a minimal, innocent murmur.

THIRD HEART SOUND

The third sound is a vibration that occurs in early diastole. It is often audible in normal children and adolescents. It is frequently found in normal phonocardiograms if they are recorded with equipment able to record low frequency vibrations. It becomes audible and is recorded by the phonocardiograph in higher frequency bands in certain groups of clinical cases.

The third sound has been related to blood flow in early diastole by several investigators. However, various theories have been advanced regarding the main structures set into vibration by this rapid flow. A motion of the ventricular wall (along with the blood) caused by the sudden inrush of blood during the early phase of diastole was suggested by Ohm, Orias and Braun-Menéndez, Wolferth and Margolies (1933), and others. The apparent coincidence of the third sound with the end of rapid filling led to the theory that this sound is produced by sudden checking of the outward motion of the ventricular wall when it reaches the limit of its passive distensibility. Gibson, T. Lewis (1925), and Dock et al., on the other hand, viewed the third sound as the result of transient closure and tension of the AV valves, caused by a temporary rebound of the blood at the end of the phase of rapid filling. A transient ventriculoatrial (VA) gradient, observed by Warren et al., seemed to support this theory. Crevasse et al., on the other hand, observed a maximal atrioventricular (AV) gradient at the time of the third sound.

According to Rushmer (1961) "the momentum of the moving mass of blood produces low frequency vibrations because the chamber walls are all relaxed. Such vibrations would be more likely to occur when the phase of rapid filling is abruptly terminated."

In conditions of *absolute diastolic overload,* a greater mass of blood enters one or both ventricles, and a moderate increase of the diastolic pressure has been accepted as the cause of the additional sound (Nixon and Wagner). Similarly, a *relative diastolic overload* (normal filling of a damaged ventricle) has been considered as an explanation for the large third sound observed in cases of myocarditis, hypertensive heart disease, or coronary heart disease with either frank or latent failure (McKusick et al., 1955). These cases often have some increase of the diastolic pressure, either in the left ventricle or in both ventricles.

The augmentation of the third sound caused by high output

is a well established clinical observation that seems to agree with theories associating the sound to flow. The accentuated third sound observed during congestive heart failure causing low output, however, is a disturbing observation. Moreover, a third heart sound has been recorded in experimental conditions independently of blood flow and valvular movement (J. R. Smith).

It has been stated that the normal third sound coincides with the peak of the wave of rapid filling that is commonly present in the ultralow (Thayer, Luisada, 1953) or low frequency tracing (Rosa, 1948) of the precordium. As it will be seen later, modern techniques show that this is not exactly true.

In recent years several studies have been undertaken to demonstrate the exact mechanism of the origin of the third sound. One of the tools used for this purpose was intracardiac phonocardiography. Crevasse et al., using the method described by Luisada and Liu (1957), studied the third sound both in dogs and in heart patients. They stated that the third sound was recorded best within the ventricles and poorly within the atria, confirming the findings of Lewis et al. (1957), Moscovitz et al. (1958), and Luisada et al. (1964).

Experimental studies were made in our laboratory by Arevalo et al. in normal dogs. The third sound was recorded best within the left ventricle, particularly near the apex in the vicinity of the left ventricular wall. A slight asynchronism between the right and left ventricular third sounds supplied evidence that the externally recorded sound was usually of left ventricular origin. It was also observed that the third sound coincided with the return to the base line of the first derivative of LV pressure (Fig. 22). In further studies correlating the third sound with volume changes of the heart, it was observed that *the sound occurred while rapid filling was still in progress.*

These experiments showed the following data:

1. There was *no* positive ventriculo-atrial gradient at the time of the third sound, a fact that is at variance with theories accepting transient AV valve tension or closure.
2. Rate-dependent changes of the second-to-third sound interval are mainly the result of changes of duration of the isovolumic

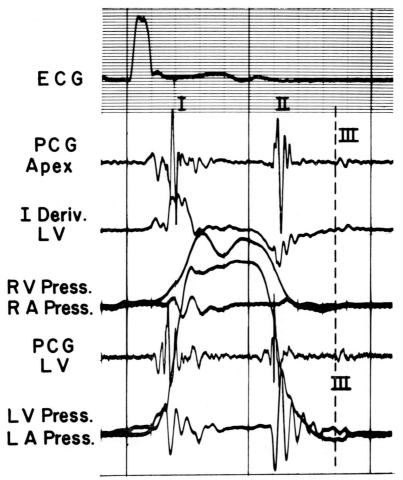

FIGURE 22. Cardiac pressures and the third heart sound. The III sound occurs when the first derivative of left ventricular pressure returns to the baseline.

relaxation phase whereas the duration of the rapid filling phase shows no significant variation.

3. A parallel prolongation of the duration of mechanical systole and of the II-III sound interval was observed during systolic overload. The release of the cause of overload (aortic obstruction) produced a reversal of this time relationship.

4. With marked aortic obstruction, the third sound may occur when ventricular pressure still exceeds atrial pressure, *a condition that excludes flow from the atrium* (Fig. 23).

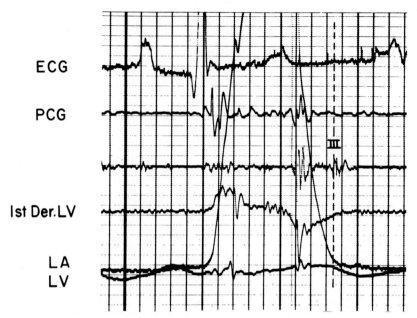

ECG

PCG

Ist Der. LV

LA
LV

FIGURE 23. The third sound can occur even when, in the presence of extreme aortic obstruction, the mitral valve cannot open. Pressure tracings and external and internal PCG during extreme overloading of the left ventricle in a dog. In the cycle shown here, a third sound occurs in the left ventricle even though no opening of the mitral valve has occurred due to high LV diastolic pressure. (From Arevalo *et al.:* J. Appl. Physiol., 1964, courtesy of the Publisher.)

These observations led to the conclusion that the third sound cannot be attributed to either blood flow or its sudden arrest. On the other hand, the time relationship of the third sound to changes in the duration of ventricular relaxation suggests a relationship between this sound and the process of myocardial relaxation itself.

The constant time coincidence of the third sound with the return to the base line of the first derivative of ventricular pressure indicates that *the third sound occurs when intraventricular volume and accommodation have reached a state of balance and intramural tension begins to rise once more.*

A possible energy source is embodied in the blood volume present in the ventricles at the time of transition from active relaxation to passive distension. Once active relaxation has ceased, each ventricle must of necessity adjust to accommodate its contained volume of blood. If such volume is minimal, the distending force and resulting vibrations would also be small. On the other hand, an increased intraventricular volume (whether the result of greater residual volume or increased filling) would increase the distending force and accentuate the third sound.

This concept seems adequate to explain the accentuated third sound in conditions with either heart failure and increased residual volume or volume overload without failure.

FOURTH HEART SOUND (ATRIAL SOUND)

A fourth sound in presystole was first described by Charcelay and by Clark.

The fourth sound is found more often in patients with delayed AV conduction, in whom greater separation between the atrial sound and the first sound makes auditory perception of the two sounds easier.

As a graphic phenomenon, the fourth sound can be found in the tracings of normal persons (especially children) as a small, low-pitched vibration. Whenever it has greater amplitude (and often a higher pitch) it is a pathologic phenomenon.

The fourth sound is heard and recorded more often than the third in cases with ischemic or hypertensive heart disease, and is also common in myocarditis, hyperthyroidism, and heart failure. The fourth sound is particularly increased in conditions of ventricular systolic overload, such as pulmonary stenosis or pulmonary hypertension (right heart) and aortic stenosis or systemic hypertension (left heart).

The same maneuvers and positions that decrease the third sound also decrease the fourth sound through the decrease of venous return, whereas vasoconstrictor drugs increase this sound. This shows the connection between the fourth sound and an absolute or relative cardiac overload. This sound has been explained as the result of *increased atrial dynamics in the presence of a decreased compliance of one of the ventricles.*

The phonocardiogram in the medium low-frequency range reveals either a diphasic or a triphasic slow wave in presystole.

Occasionally three or four small vibrations can be recorded, and sometimes the splitting of this sound can be observed. It has been stated that the fourth sound may fuse with the first sound and even occur after the Q wave of the ECG (Kincaid-Smith and Barlow, 1959). This is open to question, however, because the first sound itself starts with a slow vibration that is present even in cases of atrial fibrillation (Luisada, 1953, Counihan *et al.*) or complete AV block (Schuetz *et al.*). An exception may be represented by children or adolescents with a short P-R interval when the atrial sound may continue with the vibrations of the first sound.

Long ago, French cardiologists noted that, both in cases of atrial flutter and in cases of AV block, it was possible to hear and record additional sounds, louder in the former than in the latter. The phonocardiogram most often records only one low-pitched vibration, occasionally two (Lewis, T., 1925, Folferth and Margolies, 1940), and even three (Calo, 1950).

Since the description by T. Lewis (1925) and the study of Weitzman, the atrial sound has been considered as a complex consisting of two different components: a first group of low-amplitude, low-pitch vibrations, and a second group of larger, more rapid vibrations occuring from 50 to 90 msec. later. The first component was recorded best from the esophagus (Tequini) and was attributed to atrial contraction *per se*. The second group, best recorded over the apex, was explained as the result of either ventricular distension or tensing of the AV valves. Evidence for the latter mechanism has been claimed by some authors.

According to van der Henst and Keirsebelik, an increase of the fourth sound is the result of the exaggeration of the atrial contraction and better transmission of sound through an altered ventricular wall. Atrial hypertrophy and elevated atrial pressure have been suggested by Angley *et al.* (1960) as factors responsible for the atrial sound.

Intracardiac phonocardiography has been used for the study of the atrial sound by Moscovitz *et al.* (1958), van der Henst and Keirsebelik, and Crevasse *et al.*

In an experimental study performed in our laboratory by means of simultaneous intracardiac pressure tracings and intracardiac phonocardiograms (Muiesan *et al.*), two components were usually recorded, occasionally three (Fig. 24).

The first group of vibrations is *simultaneous with the onset of atrial contraction* and is obviously caused by it; it is recorded more frequently and with greater amplitude within the atrial chambers. The second group of vibrations occurs *shortly after atrial pressure has reached its maximum* and blood is being forced into the ventricles; it is maximal within the ventricles. Both components are greatly increased by an increase of blood flow. In some of the experiments, a brief reversal of the AV pressure gradient was noted after the end of atrial contraction and before onset of ventricular contraction. This was accompanied by a third presystolic component. In these instances, *presystolic tensing of the AV valves* seems to be responsible for the third group of vibrations.

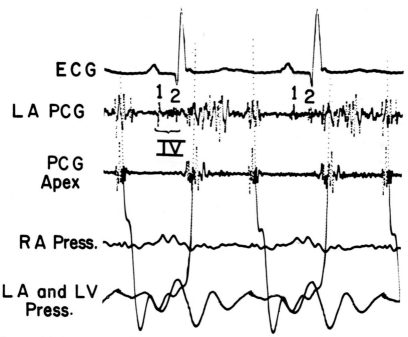

FIGURE 24. Pressure tracings and phonocardiograms of a dog. The intracardiac phonocardiogram of the left atrium (LA PCG) shows two presystolic components of the IV sound (1,2) that were not recorded from the chest wall. (From Muiesan *et al.*: Am. J. Physiol., 1961, courtesy of the Publisher.)

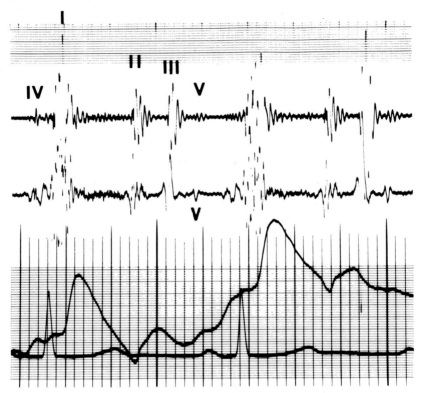

FIGURE 25. The fifth sound of the heart. Tracings recorded in a 21 year old woman with sickle cell anemia. *From above:* PCG velocity tracing (filter 50-400); PCG acceleration tracing; jugular tracing (with large carotid impact); electrocardiogram.

FIFTH HEART SOUND

The name fifth sound was given by Calo (1949) to a small, low frequency vibration that he observed in diastole after the third sound. For a long time, I have doubted the existence of this sound because one can observe two successive vibrations in early diastole that represent third sounds from the right and left ventricles that are not simultaneous. However, I have recently observed one case in which the third sound was followed 120 msec. later by another slow vibration (Fig. 25). The interval between the two was too long for admitting a double third sound and, therefore, the existence of a fifth sound should be accepted. In regard to its cause, there is no known physiologic event that

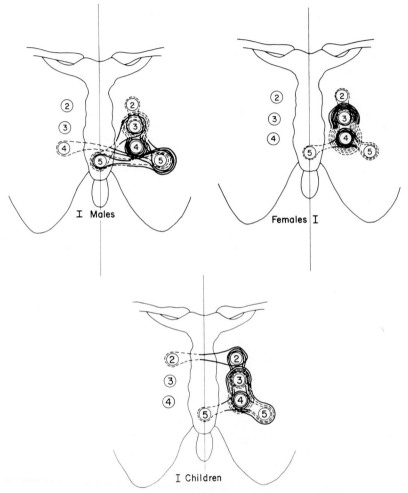

FIGURE 26. Area of greatest intensity (black line) and second best intensity (dotted line) in 10 young men, 10 young women, and 10 children for the main component of the first heart sound (I). Primary and secondary areas of intensity of each individual are connected by a loop. (From Sainani and Luisada: Am. J. Cardiol., 1967, courtesy of the Publisher.)

might cause sound in mid-diastole and we should wait for confirmation and further studies.

MAPPING OF PRECORDIUM FOR HEART SOUND AMPLITUDE

A systematic study of the amplitude of the heart sounds was made by Sainani and Luisada in 30 normal subjects. It was based

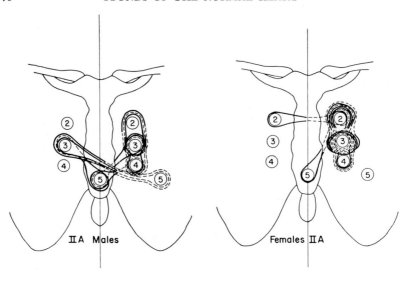

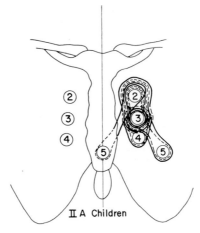

FIGURE 27. Area of greatest intensity (black line) and second best intensity (dotted line) in 10 young men, 10 young women and 10 children for the aortic component of the second heart sound (IIA). The primary and secondary areas of intensity for each individual are connected by a loop. (From Sainani and Luisada: Am. J. Cardiol., 1967, courtesy of the Publisher.)

on the graphic recording of the amplitude of the main components of the first heart sound, the aortic component of the second heart sound, and the pulmonary component of the second

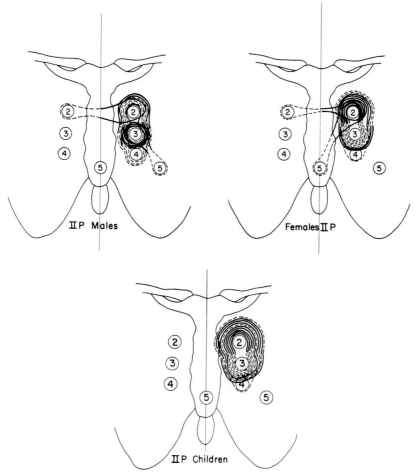

FIGURE 28. Area of greatest intensity (black line) and second best intensity (dotted line) in 10 young men, 10 young women and 10 children for the pulmonary component of the second heart sound (IIP). The primary and secondary areas of intensity for each individual are connected by a loop. (From Sainani and Luisada: Am. J. Cardiol., 1967, courtesy of the Publisher.)

heart sound. The tracings were recorded over eight precordial areas.

The *first heart sound was found generally largest over the* midprecordium (left parasternal area); exceptions were represented by a few cases having the largest first sound at the apex, at the fifth sternal or fourth right parasternal area, or even at the second right interspace. No basic difference existed in the maximal amplitude and spread of the first two components of the first sound (Fig. 26).

The *aortic component of the second heart sound was found largest* generally over the midprecordium. Exceptions were represented by a few cases having the largest aortic component over the second or fourth left parasternal interspace (Fig. 27).

The *pulmonary component of the second heart sound was generally* largest over the second left interspace (Fig. 28).

The *third and fourth sounds,* when recorded in children, had maximal amplitude in the left parasternal areas.

These data confirm a recent systematization of the auscultatory areas of the precordium but are in contrast with older views on the areas of auscultation of the heart.

Chapter 9

Murmurs and Their Mechanism

CARDIOVASCULAR murmurs are "noises" because they contain sound vibrations of different frequencies. In this sense, heart sounds also are noises. Therefore, the difference between a heart sound and a heart murmur is a clinical one.

Snaps or clicks are short series or high pitched vibrations (usually not more than 2 to 3 diphasic vibrations in the 100 to 500 hz range). (Examples: the ejection sound, the opening snap.)

Dull sounds are short series of low or medium pitched vibrations (usually not more than 1 to 2 diphasic vibrations in the 5 to 50 hz range). (Examples: the third and fourth sound.)

Normal heart sounds are longer series of vibrations, including low-medium-, and high-frequency vibrations.

Average cardiac murmurs are even longer series of vibrations. There may be predominance of either the low pitched *(rumbles)*, or the high pitched vibrations *(blowing murmurs)*. There may not be any significant predominance (outflow tract murmurs, murmur of ventricular septal defect).*

Musical murmurs represent an exception because they contain predominantly vibrations of a certain frequency; thus the observer hears a single note that repeats itself regularly and sounds "musical."

There has been an attempt to attribute most murmurs to

the fact that blood flow ceases to be laminar or streamlined and becomes *turbulent* in a certain section of the cardiovascular system because of narrowing or dilation (Rushmer). This mechanism has been questioned, however. According to McKusick, "most murmurs arise through a complex interplay of disturbed flow and the wall and other boundary structures."

Reynolds formula is of importance in application to murmurs. The Reynolds number is based on the following formula:

$$\frac{\text{Diameter of conduit} \times \text{Velocity of flow}}{\text{Kinematic viscosity of fluid}}$$

Decreased viscosity *(anemia)* is conducive to murmurs whereas increased viscosity *(polycythemia)* tends to abolish them. Local changes in diameter (narrowing of a valve, dilatation of the aorta or pulmonary artery) are common causes of murmurs. Increased velocity of blood flow or increased volume of blood flow through a vessel or valve of normal caliber is also a frequent cause of murmurs.

Loud murmurs arise more easily in soft-walled tubes rather than in rigid tubes, probably because the walls, vibrating together with the blood, have larger motions.

Murmurs result from a *pressure gradient* that generates a stream velocity sufficient to produce *vortices,* and the velocity is proportional to the square root of the pressure gradient, which in turn depends on the volume of flow per unit cross-section area of the orifice (Rodbard, 1964). A high velocity of the blood stream is often associated with a relatively small flow volume.

Eddies and *vortices* should be distinguished from turbulence and have been considered the cause of most murmurs (McDonald). The area of localized eddy formation is carried downstream not much more than 10 diameters of the flow channel

---

*The description of the composition of murmurs also applies to *thrills.* A thrill is the palpatory impression of precordial vibrations of a certain frequency and magnitude. The hand has a higher threshold in regard to magnitude, and a lower threshold in regard to frequency, in comparison with the ear. Thus, a murmur of low frequency and moderate amplitude (mitral stenosis) or a murmur of medium and high frequency and great amplitude (aortic stenosis) is easily palpated. A blowing murmur of very high frequency is usually of small magnitude and cannot be palpated. Example: murmurs of aortic or mitral insufficiency, with rare exceptions.

(Meisner and Rushmer). Thus formation of eddies is localized. This seems confirmed by the fact that the regurgitant murmur of mitral insufficiency may be large on the atrial side of the mitral valve but is largely dissipated near the posterior wall of the left atrium. The vibrations developing in a flexible structure depend much more upon the elasticity of the wall than upon the driving forces (Meisner and Rushmer).

Cavitation has been considered as a possible cause of murmurs (McKusick, Meisner and Rushmer), but seems unlikely.

Flittering, an extremely rapid opening and closure of a stenotic valve, has been suggested as the cause of a stenotic murmur (Rodbard, 1957). Although rapid vibration of the semi-rigid valve leaflets can be accepted, repeated opening and closure does not seem likely during the phase of ejection because it would be revealed by an arterial pulse tracing.

The bulk of the acoustic energy in murmurs is caused by *nearly periodic fluctuations* downstream of an obstacle, and the characteristics of this type of flow are similar to those associated with *æoliar tones* (Bruns).

The vast majority of "organic" murmurs would be the result of protuberances or wall discontinuities of the heart, valves, or larger vessels. These murmurs are intensified by a relatively small increase in the velocity of the flowing blood.

For further discussions on the origin of murmurs one should consult Allen and Mustian.

Musical murmurs have been studied in detail (McKusick *et al.,* 1955, McKusick, 1964). They can be divided into (1) the trumpet group, (2) the reed group, (3) the violin group, and (4) the flitter group.

In clinical diagnosis, both the principal location of a murmur and its preferential transmission over the chest wall are often useful in the evaluation of the origin of the murmur. Shah *et al.* (1963) have tried to classify murmurs as originating in the inflow tract or outflow tract of the left and right hearts respectively.

INFLOW TRACT MURMURS OF THE LEFT HEART (Fig. 29)

The term "inflow tract" of the left heart comprises those structures that form functionally a single chamber during the diastolic filling of the left ventricle: left atrium, left AV valve, and left ventricle. Normally, the diastolic inflow does not generate vibrations of sufficient energy for being audible; on the other hand, a turbulent flow (increased rapidity or increased quantity) or obstruction to flow will result in audible diastolic vibrations (murmur).

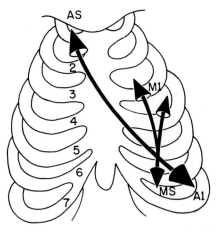

FIGURE 29. Average transmission of "inflow" and outflow" tract murmurs of the left heart. AS = aortic stenosis; AI = aortic insufficiency; MS = mitral stenosis; MI = mitral insufficiency. (From Shah *et al.*: Am. J. Cardiol., 1964, courtesy of the Publisher.)

Systolic Murmur

The murmur caused by *mitral insufficiency* may be designated as the systolic murmur of the left inflow tract. The most frequent cause of this murmur is organic mitral insufficiency (rheumatic, bacterial, or congenital). A special type of congenital lesion is found in AV communis. *Relative mitral insufficiency* may result from left ventricular enlargement with dilatation of the mitral ring and stretch of the papillary muscles. This murmur may also result from rupture or sclerosis of a papillary muscle or chorda, caused by bacterial endocarditis or myocardial infarction. The murmur caused by these conditions is preferentially located over the left ventricular and left atrial areas (Figs. 28 and 33). It is usually pansystolic but may be louder in either early systole *(decrescendo)* or in late systole *(crescendo)*. The murmur caused by papillary muscle dysfunction is more often late-systolic. It is essentially a medium and high-pitched murmur. A ruptured chorda may give rise to a *musical murmur*.

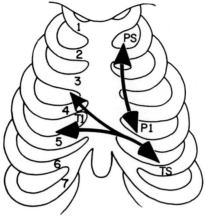

FIGURE 30. Average transmission of "inflow" and "outflow" tract murmurs of the right heart. PS = pulmonic stenosis; PI = pulmonic insufficiency; TS = tricuspid stenosis; TI = tricuspid insufficiency. (From Shah *et al.:* Am. J. Cardiol., 1964, courtesy of the Publisher.)

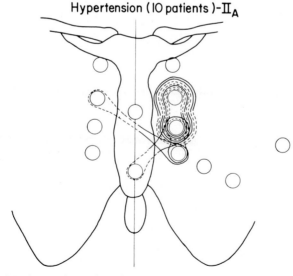

FIGURE 31. Maximum intensity of the aortic component of the second heart sound in systemic hypertension. (From Sainani *et al.:* Acta Cardiol., 1968, courtesy of the Publisher.)

Diastolic Murmur

Organic *mitral stenosis* is the most common cause of a diastolic murmur. However, it has been recognized for some time that a functional murmur resulting from increased flow across the mitral valve can be noted in the absence of organic deformity of the valve (Luisada and Pérez Montes, 1950, Luisada *et al.,* 1955, 1959). Common examples are found in mitral insufficiency and in patent ductus arteriosus with a large shunt. Rheumatic myocarditis can give rise to a similar murmur (Coombs, Zilli and Gamna). Flint described a diastolic rumble in severe aortic insufficiency, and it is still debated whether stretching of the papillary muscles causing approximation of the valve leaflets, turbulence caused by two meeting streams of blood, or a ventriculo-atrial gradient temporarily closing the mitral valve is involved.

The murmur of mitral stenosis is usually localized to the medial part of the left ventricular area and obviously commences after the opening of the mitral valve. It is usually low-pitched, rumbling, and mid-diastolic; atrial contraction accentuates the murmur in presystole, creating a high-pitched crescendo phase.

The "functional" diastolic rumble is more often mid-diastolic (starting with or after a large III sound), is recorded over a larger area than the rumble of organic stenosis, and has also often larger, low pitched vibrations.

OUTFLOW TRACT MURMURS OF THE LEFT HEART (Fig. 29)

The term "outflow tract" includes the structures that are in direct continuity during left ventricular ejection after opening of the aortic valve. These structures are the left ventricle, the aortic root, and the ascending aorta.

Systolic Murmur

A commonly recognized organic condition responsible for this murmur is *aortic valvular stenosis.* Cases of *subaortic stenosis* are being reported with greater frequency while *supravalvular stenosis* is a rare cause. Increased flow across the aortic valve may also produce this murmur. This occurs in *high output states* (anemia, thyrotoxicosis, arteriovenous fistulas, or beriberi heart), in states with *increased left ventricular ejection* (aortic insuffi-

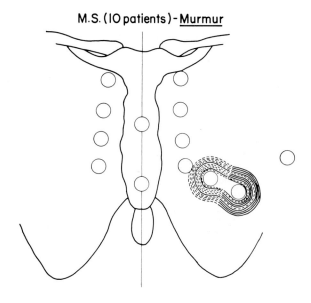

FIGURE 32. Maximum intensity of the first heart sound (A), opening snap (B), and diastolic murmur (C) in mitral stenosis. (From Sainani *et al.:* 1968, courtesy of the Publisher.)

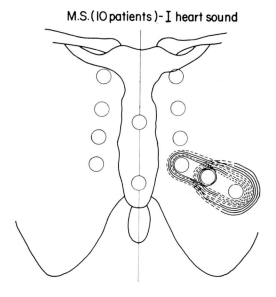

M.S. (6 patients) - O.S.

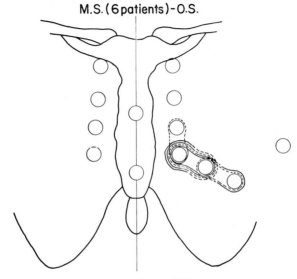

FIGURE 34B.

ciency, patent ductus arteriosus), and in cases with *dilatation of the ascending aorta* (atherosclerosis, aortitis, Marfan syndrome). The murmur usually has the maximal loudness over the second right interspace only if the aorta is dilated while it is better audible over the left ventricular area if no such dilatation is present (Figs. 29 and 34). The murmur of aortic stenosis often commences with a snapping sound after the opening of the aortic valve *(ejection sound)* and is well separated from the main body of the first heart sound. It often ends before aortic valve closure and presents a crescendo-decrescendo (diamond-shaped). It is medium and high-pitched, and is often very loud.

Diastolic Murmur

This murmur usually indicates organic aortic insufficiency caused by either deformity of the valve, its perforation, or lack of support because of an altered aortic ring. It may be caused by relative aortic insufficiency, secondary to dilatation of the aortic ring (aneurysm of the sinus of Valsalva, aortitis,* atherosclero-

---

*In these cases, dilatation of the ring and fibrotic alterations of the leaflets are often associated.

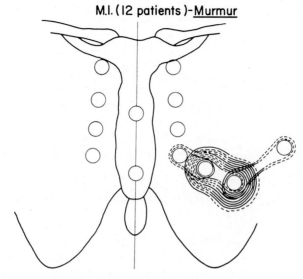

FIGURE 33. Maximum intensity of the pansystolic murmur of mitral insufficiency. (From Sainani *et al.*: Acta Cardiol., 1968, courtesy of the Publisher.)

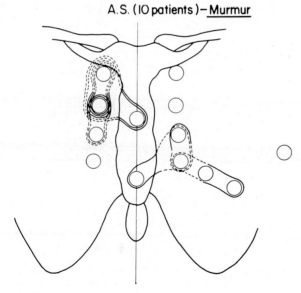

FIGURE 34. Maximum intensity of the systolic murmur of aortic stenosis. (From Sainani *et al.*: Acta Cardiol., 1968, courtesy of the Publisher.)

sis,** long-standing hypertension) or incomplete rupture of the aorta.*** This murmur is heard over both the aortic and left ventricular areas (Fig. 35). It commences early in diastole after aortic valve closure but occasionally before the second sound; it is high-pitched, soft, blowing, and is followed by a long decrescendo phase. The murmur is louder at the left of the sternum in the average case but may be louder at the right of the sternum in cases of aortic aneurysm or dilatation, Marfan syndrome, or dissecting aneurysm of the aorta (Harvey *et al.*, Sainani *et al.*, 1968).

INFLOW TRACT MURMURS OF THE RIGHT HEART

As in the left side of the heart, the inflow tract of the right heart includes the right atrium, the right AV valve, and the inflow tract of the right ventricle. These form a functionally continuous tract in diastole after the opening of the tricuspid valve. A systolic murmur of this tract would result from an incompetent tricuspid valve, whereas a diastolic murmur would be caused by either stenosis or increased flow across the valve. Inspiration, which augments venous inflow to the right heart, usually accentuates these murmurs (Rivero Carvallo).

Systolic Murmur

Organic tricuspid insufficiency is caused by a congenital deformity of the tricuspid valve in the AV communis type of defect or in Ebstein's malformation. A rheumatic lesion may occur in some cases of rheumatic valvular disease. The most common form, however, is *relative tricuspid insufficiency,* secondary to dilation and enlargement of the right ventricle and is found in severe right heart failure like that resulting from either severe mitral stenosis or pulmonary heart disease. This murmur is located over the right ventricular and right atrial areas, especially the latter (Fig. 30). It is pansystolic and is medium or high pitched.

**In atherosclerosis, lesions occurring above the ring cause lowering of one or more leaflets.

***Following dissection of the ascending aorta, the tear may close but one of the aortic leaflets is lower than normally.

Diastolic Murmur

Organic tricuspid stenosis is a possible cause of diastolic murmur. Rheumatic valvular stenosis is by no means rare while a congenital lesion is rare. On the other hand, *relative tricuspid stenosis* caused by increased and turbulent flow across the valve (atrial septal defect) is a far more common cause of this murmur. This murmur is localized to the right ventricular area (Fig. 29) and is low-pitched aid rumbling. It may be short, but occasionally one can hear a long diastolic-presystolic murmur.

OUTFLOW TRACT MURMURS OF THE RIGHT HEART (Fig. 30)

The infundibulum of the hight ventricle, the pulmonary valve, and the main pulmonary artery constitute the outflow tract of the right heart. This tract is in functional continuity during right ventricular ejection following the opening of the pulmonary valve. Either increased or accelerated flow or obstruction to flow may give rise to a systolic murmur, whereas insufficiency of the pulmonary valve would cause a diastolic murmur.

Systolic Murmurs

Organic pulmonary valvular stenosis, which is a frequent cause of systolic murmur, is most often congenital. It may be either isolated or associated with other defects. *Infundibular stenosis,* which is most frequently associated with a ventricular septal defect *(tetralogy of Fallot),* may also give rise to a similar murmur. A frequent murmur is that produced by either *accelerated or increased pulmonary flow* (anemia, beriberi heart, thyrotoxicosis, atrial septal defect, chronic cor pulmonale) or *dilatation of the pulmonary artery,* the most typical being idiopathic dilatation. A frequent variety of innocent murmurs of children is produced at this tract. The murmur is chiefly located over the pulmonary area and may extend to the right ventricular area.

Diastolic Murmur

Insufficiency of the pulmonary valve produces this diastolic murmur. Organic valvular deformity is a rare cause, whereas dilatation of the pulmonary ring is more frequent. The most common cause of this dilatation is long-standing pulmonary

hypertension, as in mitral stenosis, chronic cor pulmonale, idiopathic pulmonary hypertension, or Eisenmenger's syndrome.
This murmur is heard best over the pulmonary and right ventricular areas and starts after the pulmonary component of the
second sound.

MURMURS PRODUCED AT THE SITE OF A LEFT-TO-RIGHT SHUNT

Large abnormal shunts produce acoustic vibrations within
the recipient chamber, then emerging on the overlying surface
of the precordium. Patent ductus arteriosus, an aorto-pulmonary
septal defect, or a shunt resulting from rupture of a sinus Valsalva
give rise to a typical continuous murmur; this is maximal over
the first and second left interspaces in the former, whereas it is
usually loudest in the third left interspace in the latter. Ventricular septal defect produces a loud, long, pansystolic murmur
over the right ventricle. Atrial septal defect rarely gives rise to
an audible murmur at the site of the shunt because of both the
minimal small pressure gradient between the atria and the large
size of the defect. However, a murmur is recorded within the
right atrium.

MURMURS OF DISTAL GREAT VESSEL NARROWING

Constriction of a great vessel results in a murmur that is
loud distal to the narrowing, and of low magnitude proximal to
it. This is particularly true in *coarctation of the aorta,* where the
site of the coarctation can at times be localized by clinical
auscultation. The murmur is heard best along the descending
thoracic aorta in the left interscapulo-vertebral space. Similarly,
coarctation of the branches of the pulmonary artery results in a
murmur distal to the narrowing, which is well transmitted to the
axillæ and the back.

This dynamic interpretation serves to emphasize the fact
that a murmur is the result of abnormal flow (augmented, accelerated, obstructed, or passing through an abnormal channel)
and that, during this flow, the expelling and receiving chambers
behave like a functionally single chamber. This results in the
transmission of the murmur both to the ejecting and the receiving
chamber, though more to the latter.

Obviously, in the transmission of these vibrations from a chamber to the chest wall, other factors, such as the proximity of the area of vibration to the chest wall and the interposed tissues, are involved.

It should be kept in mind that murmurs of great magnitude may spread, first to the heart, then to the chest, and further, through the bone structures, to distant points of the body. Since the greatest magnitude of murmurs usually occurs in aortic or pulmonary stenosis, ventricular septal defect, or patent ductus arteriosus because of the dynamic energy of the chamber propelling the blood, these murmurs most commonly spread outside the conventional areas. The loud musical diastolic murmur of a ruptured or perforated aortic cusp or the musical systolic murmur caused by a ruptured chorda of the mitral valve may also be transmitted by bone structures.

MAPPING OF THE PRECORDIUM FOR MURMURS AND ABNORMAL SOUNDS

A graphic study was conducted in 54 patients by Sainani *et al.* (1968) in order to document the best locations for recording heart sounds and murmurs.

(1) The ringing second sound of systemic hypertension was generally recorded best at the left of the sternum (Fig. 31).

(2) The snapping first sound of mitral stenosis was recorded best at the apex but also over higher locations (Fig. 32A). The *opening snap* was recorded best over the lower left parasternal areas (Fig. 32B). The *mid-diastolic and presystolic murmur* was recorded best over the apex and also over a higher and more medial location (Fig. 32C).

(3) The *pansystolic murmur of mitral insufficiency* was recorded best over the apex, followed by a higher and more medial area (Fig. 33).

(4) The *diamond-shaped systolic murmur of aortic stenosis* was recorded best at the right of the sternum in one-half of the cases; over the center of the sternum, the left of the sternum, or even the apex, in the other half (Fig. 34).

(5) The *blowing diastolic murmur of aortic insufficiency*

was recorded best at the right of the sternum in syphilitic heart patients, at the left of the sternum in rheumatic heart patients (Fig. 35).

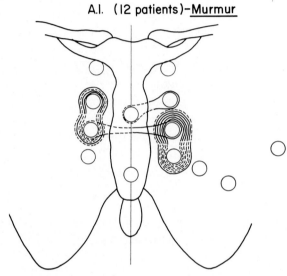

A.I. (12 patients)-<u>Murmur</u>

FIGURE 35. Maximum intensity of the diastolic murmur of aortic insufficiency. (From Sainani *et al.:* Acta Cardiol. 1968, courtesy of the Publisher.)

Chapter 10

Transmission of Sound

W E STILL lack exact quantitative data in precordial vibratory measurements, especially in regard to the magnitude of the internal vibratory energy. The central problem is the derivation of the internal force function in terms of the available network response. Although ballistocardiography has been partially successful in its attempt to assess the central force function in terms of the total body network response, a less rigorous and more practical approach is employed by phonocardiography and precordial vibrocardiography (Eddleman *et al.;* Hollis and Vidrine, Rosa, 1948, 1958, 1959; Agress *et al.;* Edson *et al.;* Harrison *et al.;* Mounsey, 1959). Because of the proximity to the source, such techniques have been useful for the empirical evaluation of the force function over the precordial area.

In order to extend the scope and value of these techniques, we need to know the attenuation properties (as a function of frequency) of the path between the heart and the external chest wall.

IMPEDANCE CHARACTERISTICS OF THE BODY NETWORK

In an effort to analyze the impedance characteristics of various components of the body network, the response of the body has been evaluated in terms of an applied steady state force function (Von Wittern, Von Gierke *et al.,* Coermann *et al.*).

The thorax is unique in that it constitutes a complex network that is loosely coupled to the internal cardioaortic network, on the one hand, and to the body network on the other.

A frequency analysis of the vibratory spectrum cannot be quantitatively correlated with the source output (the heart) without exact data on the impedance characteristics of the horax. Furthermore, if the transmission characteristics of the medium are not simple with respect to frequency, any correlation between the frequency spectrum of the chest wall vibrations and that of the actual source would be empirical.

RESPONSE CHARACTERISTICS OF THE THORACIC NETWORK

The response characteristics of the thoracic network as a whole, though a function of its individual components, cannot be directly related to that of any single component. Even though anatomic details may modify the overall response, the medium could be theoretically considered as being linear and isotropic. The relationship between input and output across such a medium might then be considered adequate for the determination of the *impedance*.

Dock found that the intensity of sound evoked by cardiac tissues subjected to a calibrated tensing force was directly related to the magnitude of the force, whereas its attenuation was directly related to the distance of the pickup from the source and to the composition of the medium. A total attenuation of 25 to 30 db was the estimated loss between source and pickup. The results of this study coincide with the findings of Bertrand *et al.*

The problem of the transfer of vibrational energy from one structure to another has been called *acoustic coupling*.

According to D. H. Lewis, resistance to motion will be determined by (1) the relationship between mass and frictional resistance, and (2) the reactance (determined by the weight of the mass and the stiffness of the surrounding structures). Both will make up the impedance to motion. At low frequencies, *stiffness* of the structures is the most important factor; at a higher frequency (the resonant frequency), the impedance is only determined by *frictional resistance;* at even higher frequencies, *reactance* again becomes a factor, and the motion of the mass decreases.

Full knowledge of the distortion of frequency and duration would require complete information of the damping characteristics of the various tissues, which is not yet available.

The transmission characteristics of the thorax have been studied in the dog by Zalter *et al.* (1963). The *frequency spectrum* of the vibrating energy presented a relative peak in the vicinity of 120 hz and then a nearly constant decline (vibrations between 1 and 30 hz were not recorded). A *transmission* loss of 20 to 40 db for the parasternal areas was found in the dog in the supine position. However, it should be noted that this loss was based on artificial vibrations introduced in the right atrium.

This study has been again undertaken by means of a new calibrated phonocardiographic system by MacCanon *et al.* The heart sounds were measured on the skin of the chest, then on muscle, pleura, lung, and pericardium. Analysis of the data showed a *loss in sound intensity level of approximately 20 db from the myocardium to the chest surface.*

In other experiments of our laboratory, one SF1 was placed within the left ventricle, another under the skin overlaying the apex (following injection of 5 cc of saline solution) or in the pericardial sac (following injection of 20 cc of saline solution). The tip of the second catheter was always directed towards the heart. A similar pattern of vibrations between left ventricular cavity and pericardial sac was noted, and also between left ventricular cavity and subcutaneous tissues. The transmission loss for the first sound between left ventricle and subcutaneous tissues was 59 db at 10 hz and 27 db at 100 hz with an average of 34 db. The loss would be greater for man because of the greater distance between heart and chest wall.

On the surface of the body, the *velocity of conduction* of heart sounds is about 15 meters per second for frequencies of 100 hz, and seems to increase with the square root of the frequency (Faber and Burton).

Faber studied the damping of frequencies from 50 to 400 hz in the soft tissues and ribs of man. For frequencies under 100

---

*Recent experiments have extended Zalter's data to the 5-30 hz range. Relative peaks have been recorded at 8 and 24 hz with the maximum power at about 8 hz. The shape of the power spectrum did not remain constant when recorded at various layers from the pleura to the skin.

hz, the chest wall appeared to be homogenous. For frequencies above 100 hz, the damping was much less for transmission over the sternum than for transmission elsewhere on the precordium.

It seems that sound travels from the heart to one or more points of the chest wall, and from there it travels along straight lines, especially along bones. This seems particularly true for frequencies above 100 hz and may not be true for lower frequencies (Faber).

There are many interfaces between the source of heart sounds and the sound detector. The material of each interface (e.g., lung tissue, fat, pleura, skin, bone) is likely to have a different acoustic impedance. Therefore, it is likely that the wave pattern of sound energy which is transmitted from the inside of the body to the outside will have a different form from the original. Moreover, the modifications imposed by these interfaces may be different when sound is transmitted from the outside to the inside in comparison with the normal transmission. Certainly the distribution of sound energy, both as a function of frequency and of position, will not be the same in both directions. Therefore, care must be taken when transmission measurements are performed with an external generator and an intracardiac or esophageal microphone, to correct for the scattering of the sound and for the spatial displacement of the detector.

TRANSMISSION OF MURMURS

Considerable discussions have arisen about transmission of murmurs. Intracardiac phonocardiography has confirmed that murmurs are transmitted by the blood in the direction toward which it is moving at the time of their production. On the other hand, murmurs are transmitted from the heart and great vessels to the chest wall. Once their vibrations have reached the bony structures, they will be carried by bone to a great distance if they have great magnitude (Levine and Likoff).

DYNAMIC RANGE OF AMPLITUDE

The dynamic range of amplitude covered by the frequency spectrum over a band of ten octaves (i.e., 1 to 1,000 hz) amounts grossly to 120 db (assuming a theoretical overall sloping amplitude of 12 db per octave) or 40 db per decade.

Heintzen and Victor introduced a phonocatheter into the cardiac chambers and applied a sound generator to the surface of the chest. The mean level of intensity of the collected signal was a function of the distance between the generator and the collector of sound. Thus, different locations of the generator gave signals of different magnitude according to their distance from the heart. The same is probably true when sound travels in the opposite direction, i.e., from the heart to the chest wall.

Feruglio, experimenting with an intracardiac sound generator in man, found more marked attenuation for frequencies below 100 hz and above 400 hz, the best conduction being between 150 and 350 hz. Sound seemed to be better transmitted in the female than in the male thorax, especially in the 150 to 200 hz range. Deep inspiration caused an attenuation of about 50 per cent, and expiration caused an increase of about 15 per cent over apnea or quiet respiration. Sounds were attenuated most when originating in the right and left pulmonary arteries and attenuated least when originating in the right atrium and main pulmonary artery; they were well conducted from the right ventricle to the chest wall.

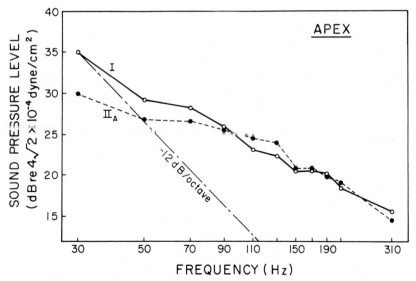

FIGURE 36. Average slope of attenuation with frequencies of the first heart sound at the apex in 11 normal young men (velocity tracing).

The relative magnitude of the heart sounds at various frequencies was studied by Sakai *et al.* in 11 normal young men over three areas of the precordium by using our new calibrated system. The average slope of attenuation for *the first heart sound* was found to be −6.5 db per octave at the apex and −7.5 db per octave at the midprecordium (Fig. 36). A slower decline was found for *the second heart sound* as the average slope of attenuation of *the aortic component* at the second left interspace was −6 db per octave up to 80 hz and no slope existed between 80 and 140 hz (Fig. 37). The *pulmonary component* of the second sound at the second left interspace had an overall slope of −3.5 db per octave (Fig. 37). A relative "peaking" was found in all subjects at different frequencies with the first heart sound usually peaking at lower frequency than the second (Fig. 38). Marked variability existed in the slope of attenuation and in the relative peaking between the various subjects.

By comparing these curves of amplitude versus frequency with the attenuation curve of 12 db/octave that had been considered typical, we can see that *the heart sounds become smaller*

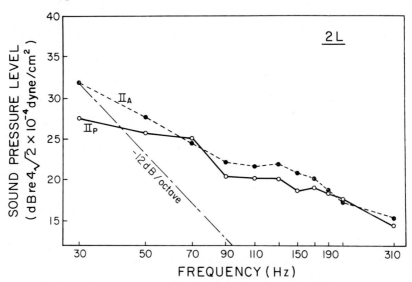

FIGURE 37. Average slope of attenuation with frequency of the two components of the second heart sound at the second left interspace in 11 normal young men (velocity tracing).

with increasing frequency but much less than the 12 db/octave curve. Therefore, current phonocardiographs which have an automatic gain of 12 db/octave will tend to overemphasize the

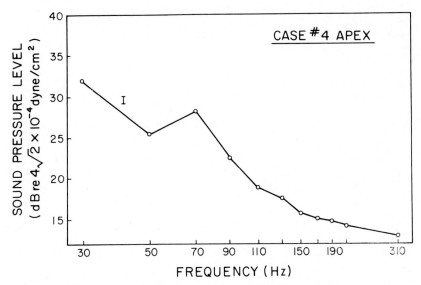

FIGURE 38. Relative peaking of the heart sounds in two normal individuals (velocity tracings). (A) Apex; (B) Midprecordium.

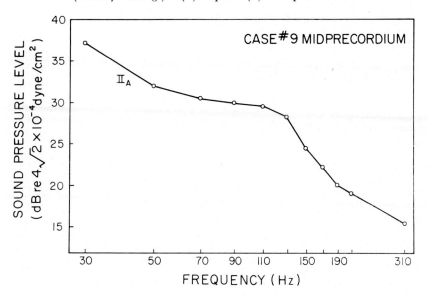

sounds in the high frequency bands. Moreover, as such auto-matic gain cannot take into account the relative peaking, it would tend to over- or under-amplify certain bands in the various individuals. The "inverse law of the square" (i.e., −12 db/octave) was based on the assumption that the sound gen-erator (heart) would originate vibrations of the same power at all frequencies. The fact that the attenuation of sounds with increasing frequency does not coincide with such a physical law can be explained in two ways: (1) The heart as a sound generator creates vibrations of various frequencies according to its own characteristics; some are larger than when a single fre-quency is experimentally generated. (2) The attenuation caused by tissue transmission and possible resonance may tend to em-phasize certain frequencies.

Part IV

AUSCULTATION

Chapter 11

The Areas of Auscultation

THE CONVENTIONAL designations of mitral, tricuspid, aortic, and pulmonary areas of auscultation (Fig. 39) have been used in textbooks, as well as in clinical descriptions, for a century or more. Probably more than one author was responsible for their description, which developed through successive steps.

Reference to heart sounds was made by Harvey and later by Morgagni. However, no further mention was made for half a century. With the introduction of the stethoscope by Laennec, cardiovascular sounds and murmurs were described but incomplete knowledge of cardiovascular physiology limited at first the accuracy of their interpretation. In 1833, the sounds supposedly arising in the right heart chambers were differentiated from those of the left heart chambers (Bertin). In 1847, Valentin described the points on the precordium where the heart sounds had their maximal intensity. In 1857, the murmurs of mitral, tricuspid, and pulmonary valvular lesions were well appreciated (Bamberger). In 1884, four auscultatory areas (mitral, tricuspid, pulmonary, and aortic) had been already accepted, and were described in Bramwell's textbook.

It is surprising that the location and interpretation of these areas, empirically selected on the basis of correlation between the location of a murmur and the finding of a diseased valve at necropsy, found little challenge until recent years.

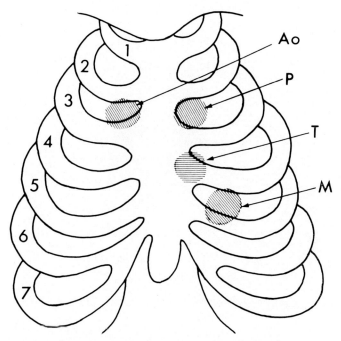

FIGURE 39. Conventional areas of auscultation.

A revision of the areas and a different interpretation of their meaning was suggested by the author with Shah and Slodki (1964). Our experience with intracardiac, epicardial, and external phonocardiograms has led to the growing conviction that the locations and designations of the areas of auscultation should be restated in terms of physiologic principles. Moreover, demonstration that the heart sounds arise in various structures and not only in the limited area of a valve (Chap. 8) required a different concept for the understanding of these areas.

It was proposed to rename the areas according to the physiologic chamber or unit in which a given sound or murmur is best recognized by intracardiac phonocardiography.

It was proposed to divide the thorax for the purpose of auscultation and phonocardiography into seven areas as follows: (1) left ventricular, (2) right ventricular, (3) left atrial, (4) right atrial, (5) aortic, (6) pulmonary, and (7) descending thoracic aortic area (Figs. 40-43).

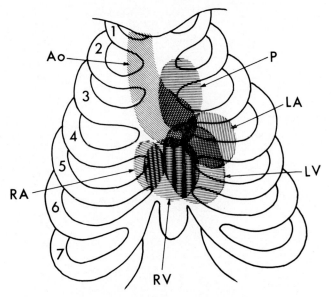

FIGURE 40. Revised areas of auscultation in the average normal heart.

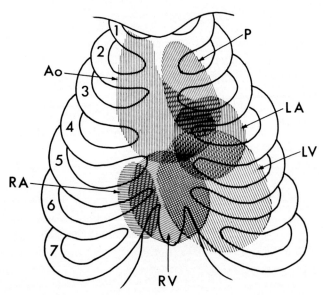

FIGURE 41. Revised areas of auscultation in cases with severe left ventricular enlargement.

LEFT VENTRICULAR AREA

The *apical area* (once called "mitral area") is the best location, not only for the murmur of mitral stenosis or insufficiency (especially the latter) but also for other acoustic phenomena that are unrelated to the mitral valve, such as the left ventricular third sound (left ventricular gallop), the left-sided fourth sound (left atrial gallop), and the aortic component

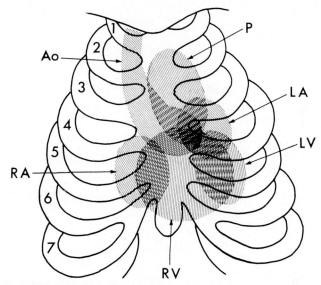

FIGURE 42. Revised areas of auscultation in cases with severe right ventricular enlargement.

of the second sound. Moreover, the murmurs of aortic stenosis* and insufficiency (especially the latter) are often heard well in this area.

Previous work (Di Bartolo *et al.*, Shah *et al.*, 1963) had demonstrated that the major rapid components of the first heart sound are best recorded within the left ventricular cavity and over the surface of the left ventricle. Graphic studies of the author with Bernstein and with Sainani demonstrated that the first heart sound is usually larger over the third left interspace than at the apex (Fig. 26). It is reasonable, therefore, to desig-

---

*The murmur caused by subaortic (muscular) stenosis is heard chiefly in this location.

nate this area as *left ventricular* rather than mitral. It is understandable that the left ventricle cannot be, and is not, a pinpointed location but a diffuse area around and above the apex, extending to the fourth and fifth left interspaces about 2 cm medially, and to the anterior axillary line laterally. In cases of left ventricular enlargement, the area would extend more medially, whereas in cases of right ventricular enlargement it would be shifted more to the left.*

In conclusion, it is suggested not only to rename the mitral area as the *left ventricular area* but also to point out that it is both larger and more variable in location than previously admitted.

RIGHT VENTRICULAR AREA

A similar case can be made for renaming the so-called *tricuspid area* as *the right ventricular area*. In this location are heard, not only the murmurs of tricuspid stenosis and insufficency, but also the right ventricular third sound (right ventricular gallop), the right atrial fourth sound (right atrial gallop), and the murmurs of pulmonary insufficiency and ventricular septal defect.

In our experience, as well as in that of others, these vibrations are normally well recorded within the cavity of the right ventricle. The murmur of tricuspid insufficiency, though best recorded in the right atrium, is also well recorded in the right ventricle. This area would then include the lower part of the sternum and the fourth and fifth interspaces, 2 to 4 cm to the left, and 2 cm to the right, of the sternum. This area may extend to the point of maximal impulse in the presence of severe right ventricular enlargement because in such cases the apex is formed by the right ventricle. Casual designation of the area coinciding with the apex beat as "the mitral area" has resulted in the past in confusion of the murmurs of tricuspid insufficiency or stenosis with those of mitral insufficiency or stenosis.

LEFT ATRIAL AREA

In normal subjects, only small vibrations coinciding with the

---

*This had been suggested by Rivero Carvallo and Garza de los Santos. Their calling "real apex" the actual left ventricular area of a patient with mitral and tricuspid valve disease is, however, confusing.

heart sounds are recorded within the atria by intracardiac phonocardiograms. In cases of mitral insufficiency, however, the lower part of the left atrial cavity is the ideal location for recording the typical systolic murmur. Even though the murmur is maximal in the left atrium, it is also recorded in the left ventricle (especially near the AV valve) and is both well heard (Lian) and recorded in the esophagus (Taquini, Miller and Groedel, Pintor *et al.*). This finding accounts for the radiation of this murmur to the left axilla, and occasionally to the back in the left interscapulovertebral area (Lian and Dang van Chung). It is not unusual to hear and record well either a mitral opening snap or a mitral systolic murmur in the third left interspace. The proximity of the left auricular appendage with this space may explain these findings.

Based on anatomic correlations, the *left atrial area* would be located above the apex extending to the left axilla, and occasionally to the area between the left scapula and the vertebral column. Caceres has suggested a "left atrial area" above the left ventricular. However, an area to the left and slightly above the apex seems to be generally the best for hearing and recording the murmur of mitral insufficiency. Certain exceptions should be kept in mind: (a) a lesion of the posterior leaflet of the mitral valve often causes a systolic murmur this is loudest over the II-III intercostal spaces; (b) a lesion of the anterior leaflet often causes a systolic murmur that is projected posteriorly toward the spine.

RIGHT ATRIAL AREA

Surface landmarks for the right atrial chamber normally extend from 1 to 2 cm to the right of the sternum in the fourth and fifth interspaces. In the presence of tricuspid insufficiency (organic or relative), the right atrium is considerably enlarged and its surface projection will extend to and beyond the right midclavicular line. This in fact is the area of radiation of the murmur of tricuspid insufficiency. It should be designated, therefore, as the *right atrial area*.

AORTIC AREA

The aortic component of the second heart sound and the murmurs of aortic valve defects are often well heard at the third left interspace (Erb's point). This area has been called the *auxiliary aortic area.* In our experience, however, the third left interspace is frequently more revealing than the second right interspace (so-called *aortic area*). This is partly explained by the anatomic proximity of the aortic valve to the third left interspace and by the absence of a thick overlying pulmonary cushion, in contrast with the second right interspace. This fact has been documented in our laboratory by graphic studies with Krol and with Sainani. The aortic component of the second sound proved to be larger at the left than at the right of the sternum, not only in normal subjects (Fig. 28), but also in the great majority of hypertensive patients (Fig. 31). In cases with dilatation of the ascending aorta, however, the manubrium of the sternum or the second right interspace may be more revealing because the dilated vessel is in close proximity of the chest wall and transmits well both the second sound and the murmurs. This fact has been documented by Harvey *et al.* Auscultation at the *suprasternal notch* (corresponding to the aortic arch) was advocated by me (1937) and by Lian (1948) in cases of aortic stenosis or insufficiency.

Therefore, the term *aortic area* should be applied to the aortic root and the ascending aorta rather than to the valve itself. The vibrations heard best at this location and detected by intravascular phonocardiograms include the murmurs caused by aortic stenosis, aortic insufficiency, augmented flow across the aorta or dilatation of the ascending aorta, and abnormalities of the arteries of the neck, as well as the aortic ejection sound and the aortic component of the second heart sound.

This area is formed by the third left interspace near the left sternal border (often including part of the second left interspace), and extends across the sternum to the first, second, and third right interspaces near the right sternal border; it may include the right sternoclavicular joint and the suprasternal notch.

PULMONARY AREA

The term *pulmonary area* should refer to the pulmonary artery rather than to the pulmonary value, as in the case of the aorta. The murmurs of pulmonary stenosis and insufficiency, the murmur caused by increased flow or dilatation of the pulmonary artery, the pulmonary ejection sound, and the pulmonary component of the second sound are usually heard best in the second left interspace but also often in the third. These vibrations can be well recorded as a rule in the intravascular phonocardiogram of the main pulmonary artery. The murmur of patent ductus arteriosus is usually recorded best in the left pulmonary artery and within the ductus itself. This explains the frequent high location of such a murmur, which is heard and recorded best in the first left space just below the clavicle.

The pulmonary area has its center in the second left interspace near the sternal border; it extends upward to the first space below the clavicle and to the left sternoclavicular joint, and downwards to the third left interspace near the sternal margin. This area may also extend posteriorly at the level of the fourth and fifth dorsal vertebræ about 2 to 3 cm to either side of the spine.

AREA FOR THE DESCENDING THORACIC AORTA

Routine auscultation and phonocardiography should also

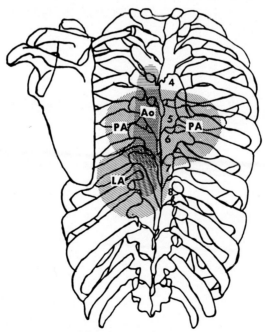

FIGURE 43. Revised areas of auscultation on the posterior aspect of the thorax.

cover the area corresponding to the *descending thoracic aorta.* This area is most revealing in cases of coarctation of the aorta (congenital or acquired) and aortic aneurysms even though a good murmur can be heard over this area also in cases of aortic stenosis. This area is located over the dorsal spine (from the second to the tenth dorsal vertebra) and would extend 2 to 3 cm to the left of the midline (Fig. 43).

Because the presence of chamber enlargement is not always obvious, it is advisable to refer the acoustic events to a given anatomic location over the chest (e.g., fourth left interspace near the sternal edge or sixth left interspace at the anterior axillary line, etc.), a procedure that is similar to that advocated by the International Committee for Standardization of Phonocardiography.

ADDITIONAL VASCULAR AREAS

Numerous other areas may be considered whenever altered vessels cause murmurs. They are the *right* and *left carotid areas,* the *abdominal aortic area,* the *flanks* (for the renal arteries), the *thyroid,* and the *femoral areas.* The venous hum is usually recorded best over the jugular bulb, just above the right clavicle.

Chapter 12

Glossary

THE *Bethesda Conferences* of the American College of Cardiology and American Heart Association* have tried to create a Standard Glossary of Cardiological Terms so that a unified terminology can be used by physicians. In doing this, the Committee has recognized that no single set of definitions is acceptable to every physician. The following definitions represent a compromise between the "auscultators" and the "phonocardiographers."

*Published in the *JAMA, 200:1041*, 1967 (Part I) and the *Am. J. Cardiol., 21:273*, 1968 (Part II).

HEART SOUNDS

Heart Sounds: These are discrete, relatively short, auditory vibrations of varying intensity (loudness), frequency (pitch), quality, and duration. Heart sounds are produced by hemodynamic events. They are of shorter duration than murmurs.

First Heart Sound: The first heart sound, which indicates the onset of ventricular systole on auscultation, coincides with the apex impulse and slightly precedes the carotid pulse.

Second Heart Sound: The second heart sound, which indicates the onset of diastole on auscultation, occurs at the end of ventricular contraction. This sound is usually of shorter duration and higher frequency than the first heart sound. By terminating the shorter pause, it allows auscultatory definition of systole and diastole during sinus rhythm.

111

Third Heart Sound: The third heart sound is low pitched and occurs in early diastole after the second heart sound (or in mid-diastole if there is a rapid heart rate). It occurs in healthy persons (physiologic third sound) or in disease states (ventricular or early diastolic sound). At times, a short outward movement of the chest wall can be palpated in diastole at the same time as this sound.

Fourth Heart Sound: The fourth heart sound (atrial sound) is a low frequency sound occurring in presystole shortly before the first heart sound. This sound can be heard in normal healthy subjects, particularly in children, or may occur in disease states (atrial or presystolic sound).

Intensity (Loudness): The terms used for grading intensity of heart sounds include faint, normal, or loud (accentuated).

Frequency (Pitch): The predominant frequency of heart sounds varies from high to low as determined by auscultation.

Quality: Abnormal heart sounds may sometimes have a peculiar tonal effect, best characterized by a descriptive term, such as muffled, snapping, or tambour-like.

Splitting: Either the first or the second heart sound or both may contain two audible components. Splitting of the first heart sound may be heard in healthy persons. The first and second components of the first heart sound are sometimes referred to as "mitral" and "tricuspid," respectively.

Splitting of the second heart sound is commonly heard in healthy persons during inspiration and generally decreases or disappears during expiration. Physiologic splitting is sometimes heard better with the patient in the sitting position. The first and second components of the second heart sound are commonly referred to as aortic and pulmonary, respectively. Splitting of the second heart sound which is not physiologic usually indicates cardiac disease and includes: (1) unusually wide splitting on inspiration, which persists during expiration; (2) wide splitting that varies only very slightly with respiration (*fixed or relatively fixed splitting*), and (3) splitting that appears or increases on expiration (*reversed or paradoxic splitting*).

Opening Snap: The opening snap is a high frequency sound occurring shortly after the second heart sound but before the third heart sound.

Pericardial Knock: The pericardial knock sound is a high pitched sound occurring shortly after the second heart sound in patients with constrictive pericarditis.

Systolic Sounds (Clicks): These sounds are of high frequency and short duration, and occur in early, mid- or late systole. The term *ejection sound* (or click) is used for the early systolic sound. A *late systolic sound* occurs during late systole before the second heart sound.

Triple Rhythm: This term refers to the cadence of the two normal heart sounds plus either the third or the fourth sound (or their summation) ; it is more common with rapid heart rate. In the past, it was called *gallop rhythm* whenever clinical evidence indicated an abnormal mechanism.

Quadruple Rhythm: This term refers to the cadence of the two normal heart sounds plus both the third and the fourth sounds; it is more common with slow heart rate.

HEART MURMURS

Murmur: A murmur is a relatively prolonged series of auditory vibrations of varying intensity (loudness) , frequency (pitch) , quality, configuration, and duration. The murmur is produced by structural changes and/or hemodynamic events in the heart or blood vessels.

Systolic Murmur: The systolic murmur begins with or after the time of the first heart sound and ends at or before the time of the second heart sound.

Diastolic Murmur: The diastolic murmur begins with or after the time of the second heart sound and ends at or before the time of the first heart sound.

Continuous Murmur: The murmur begins in systole and continues without interruption through the time of the second heart sound into all or part of diastole.

Intensity (Loudness): Murmurs, both systolic and diastolic, vary from grade 1 to grade 6. A grade 1 murmur is so faint that it can be heard only with special effort. A grade 2 murmur is faint but can be recognized readily. A grade 3 murmur is moderately loud. A grade 4 murmur is very loud. A grade 5 murmur is extremely loud. A grade 6 murmur is exceptionally loud and is heard with the stethoscope just removed from contact with the chest.

Frequency (Pitch): The predominant frequency band of the murmur varies from high to low as determined by auscultation.

Quality: The peculiar tonal effect of a murmur is best characterized by a descriptive term such as whooping, squeaky, musical, blowing, grunting, buzzing, scratchy, harsh (rough), rumbling.

Configuration (Shape)

Crescendo: The intensity (loudness) of the murmur increases progressively.

Decrescendo: The intensity (loudness) of the murmur decreases progressively.

Crescendo-Decrescendo (Diamond-Shaped): The intensity (loudness) of the murmur increases and then decreases.

Plateau (Sustained): The intensity (loudness) of the murmur remains relatively constant throughout.

Duration: A long murmur occupies all or almost all of systole or diastole. A short murmur occupies a brief period of systole or diastole.

CLASSIFICATION OF MURMURS

Systolic Murmurs

The murmurs should be characterized according to their time of onset and termination, as early systolic, mid systolic, late systolic, or holosystolic (pansystolic).

(a) Early Systolic Murmur: The early systolic murmur begins at the time of the first heart sound and ends before or about the middle of systole.

(b) Late Systolic Murmur: The late systolic murmur begins about the middle of systole and ends at the time of the second heart sound.

(c) Mid Systolic Murmur: The mid systolic murmur begins clearly after the first heart sound and ends clearly before the second heart sound. These murmurs may be separated into those which end before the first or aortic component of the second heart sound and those which end before the second or pulmonary component. Left-sided mid systolic murmurs end before the aortic component of the second heart sound, and right-sided mid systolic murmurs end before the pulmonary component.

(d) Holosystolic Murmur: The holosystolic (pansystolic) murmur begins with the first heart sound, occupies all of systole, and ends with the second heart sound. Left-sided holosystolic murmurs end with the aortic component of the second heart sound, and right-sided holosystolic murmurs end with the pulmonary component of the second heart sound.

Diastolic Murmurs

The diastolic murmurs are described according to their time of onset.

(a) Early Diastolic Murmur: The early diastolic murmur begins with either the aortic or pulmonary component of the second heart sound.

(b) Mid Diastolic Murmur: The mid diastolic murmur begins clearly after the second heart sound.

(c) Late Diastolic Murmur: The late diastolic or pre-systolic murmur is confined to the period immediately before the first heart sound.

The terms "heart sounds" and "heart murmurs," are currently employed to describe the vibrations detected by auscultation of the chest wall. The same terms were applied to vibrations of the chest wall recorded by a phonocardiograph.

Technological advances in recent years have enabled us to record vibrations within the heart and vessels by using intra-cardiac detectors. These vibrations have also been called "heart sounds" and "heart murmurs," even though they may not correspond exactly to the vibrations which are externally recorded because the process of transmission through intervening tissues necessarily modifies the vibrations.

The thorax is composed of "soft" tissues, such as the lungs, fat, and skin, and "hard" tissues, such as bone. These tissues absorb, reflect, and transmit acoustical vibrations, such as the sounds and murmurs produced by the cardiohemic system. The amount of tissue, its shape, and its location will determine in what manner it will modify the sounds which traverse it by absorbing or reflecting the energy.

Therefore, sounds and murmurs recorded at the surface of the chest have undergone modification, and thus are not identical to those produced within the heart.

Since these two kinds of detection procedures give different results, we feel that it is incorrect to call the results by the same name. For this reason, we propose that the externally recorded vibrations, which are traditionally called heart sounds and murmurs, continue to be termed as *sounds* and *murmurs,* whereas the internally detected vibrations should be called *cardiac vibrations.* In this sense the term "Intracardiac Phonocardiogram" could be changed to "Intracardiac Vibrocardiogram" or more simply *vibrocardiogram.*

This change would serve at least two useful purposes:

1. It would simplify the terminology;
2. It would help us to remember that there is a modification of the energy as it is transmitted through the chest.

Chapter 13

Most Significant Auscultatory Findings

ACCEPTED FACTS REGARDING HEART SOUNDS

THE TWO main heart sounds (the first and the second) were described by Laennec and were confirmed by all subsequent observers. The normal third sound was described by Obrastzow, Einthoven, Gibson, Hirschfelder, and Thayer. The fourth sound was first heard by Charcelay in a heart patient, and was then confirmed by other observers. Houssay mentioned four normal heart sounds (1936).

It is classic to admit certain facts regarding heart sounds.

The *first sound* is generally louder over the left ventricular area (especially over the midprecordium); the second sound is usually louder over the aortic and pulmonary areas (base). The reasons for these facts are inherent in the mechanism of production of the two heart sounds as well as in their transmission to the chest wall.

The *first sound* is a long noise of lower tonality; the second sound is shorter and sharper.

The *first sound* may be *closely split* in normal adolescents or young people in the third or fourth left interspace close to the sternum (Erb's point). This splitting is not influenced by respiration.

The *first sound* often has a *decreased loudness* in myocarditis.

117

myocardial infarct, myocardial fibrosis, hypothyroidism, mitral insufficiency, aortic insufficiency, and pericarditis with effusion. It often has an increased loudness in mitral stenosis, systemic hypertension, and hyperthyroidism.

The *second sound* is frequently *split* in normal children and young people; the best area for hearing this splitting is the third left interspace, close to the sternum (Erb's point). This splitting is usually heard best at the end of inspiration and may disappear in expiration.

The *second sound* has an *increased loudness of the aortic component* in systemic hypertension, coarctation of the aorta, or aortitis; a *decreased loudness* of this component occurs in aortic stenosis where the aortic component may be so delayed that it follows the pulmonary component, thereby resulting in reverse (or paradoxical splitting). The *second sound* has an *increased loudness of the pulmonary component* in pulmonary hypertension, primary or secondary. (In these cases the pulmonary component can be heard even at the apex.) A *decreased loudness* of this component occurs in pulmonary stenosis; the pulmonary component is not only smaller but also delayed, causing a wider splitting.

The *second sound* has a wider, *fixed splitting* in conditions presenting a diastolic overload of the right heart like atrial septal defect. The word "fixed" implies that respiratory variations are minimal or absent. Such wide splitting is also heard in mature adults who otherwise would have a single second sound or an extremely close splitting. A fixed splitting is also found in right bundle branch block as a result of the delay of the right ventricular contraction and thus of the pulmonary component. On the contrary, cases with left bundle branch block may present such a delay of the aortic component as to cause reverse splitting. Normal children may occasionally have a fixed splitting in the supine position while normal, inspiratory splitting is present when they are sitting or standing.

The *third sound* is normal in children or adolescents; it is heard as a dull sound of poor intensity, mostly over the left ventricular area (apex). It may become louder, and it may be audible over either the left or right ventricular areas in cases with ventricular overload, myocarditis, tachycardia, or heart failure. According to an older description, it is then called "ventricular gallop."

The *fourth sound (atrial sound)* is seldom heard in normal hearts (though it can be recorded). In cases with Grade 1 AV block, occasionally a low grade, faint, muffled sound precedes the first sound. A fourth sound may be audible over either the left (more common) or the right ventricular area (less common) in cases with ventricular overload, myocarditis, tachycardia, atrial flutter, complete or incomplete AV block. It is then called "atrial gallop" in reference to the mechanism of origin and not to the area of audition.

A slightly different type of extra-sound has been called "summation gallop" because it results from the summation of the third with the fourth sound. This is particularly encountered in cases with tachycardia and Grade 1 AV block having dynamic alterations that increase both the third and the fourth sounds.

An *early-systolic snap or click* can be heard over either the pulmonary (pulmonary ejection sound) or the aortic area (aortic ejection sound). These snaps are caused by either an increased loudness of the third component of the first sound (in case of the aorta) or a new sound of equivalent significance but not usually present (in the case of the pulmonary artery). Each can be found in cases with dilatation of the vessel or narrowing of the aortic or pulmonary valve (usually with poststenotic dilatation). It is most likely caused by a vibration of the vascular wall with the blood it contains (possible also of the valvular apparatus) at the beginning of ejection.

A *midsystolic or late-systolic* snap can be caused by either extra-cardiac factors (pericardial adhesions) or vibrations of a mitral leaflet (in cases with mitral insufficiency).

A *diastolic snap or click* can be heard in fourth left interspace close to the sternum, over the entire precordium. This is the *mitral opening snap,* which is most often heard in mitral stenosis. Occasionally, it can be heard also in cases of diastolic overload of the left heart (mitral insufficiency, patent ductus arteriosus).

A *tricuspid opening snap* is audible over the right ventricular area in cases of tricuspid stenosis. It can be recorded (an oc-casionally heard) also in cases of diastolic overload of the right ventricle (tricuspid insufficiency, atrial septal defect, ventricular septal defect).

DESCRIPTION OF MURMURS

Murmurs are a significant finding of auscultation.

A description of murmurs that has become popular divides the murmurs in *ejection murmurs* and *regurgitant murmurs*. This terminology cannot be encouraged because it already im-plies a recognition of the mechanism of the murmur, which is not always possible.

The *murmur of AV valve insufficiency* is blowing, prolonged, and soft; it may be either in decrescendo or pansystolic, and is occasionally in crescendo.* Whereas the murmur of mitral in-sufficiency is maximal over the left ventricular area (fourth or fifth left intercostal space) and is audible at the left atrial area (left axilla), that of tricuspid insufficiency is maximal over the right ventricular area (third or fourth left or right intercostal space) and is still audible over the right precordium.

*The "shape" of murmurs is well revealed by phonocardiography.

An *early-systolic murmur in decrescendo* typically obscures the I heart sound while the II heart sound is well heard because it follows the end of the murmur. A *pansystolic murmur* typically obscures both heart sounds because it lasts throughout ventricular systole and may even "spill" into early diastole.* A *late systolic murmur in crescendo* typically obscures the II sound and may "spill" into early diastole while the first sound is clearly heard. Inspiration or inspiratory apnea increases the loudness of the tri-cuspid murmur but decreases that of the mitral murmur.

*Occasionally, the murmur of mitral insufficiency is reinforced in mid or late systole by a louder, musical phase. This phenomenon, called *systolic whoop*, still has no adequate explanation.

The *murmur of AV valve stenosis* is a typical, low-pitched rumble that acquires higher pitch and greater loudness in pre-systole (if there is sinus rhythm). In mitral stenosis, it is heard best in the fourth left intercostal space, halfway between the apex and the sternal border, as documented by Sainani with the author. In tricuspid stenosis, it is heard best in either the third left intercostal space or the third right intercostal space according to the size and position of the heart (right ventricular area). This murmur often becomes louder in inspiration or inspiratory apnea.

The *murmur of the semilunar valves stenosis* is probably the loudest of all. It is harsh, starts a bit after the first sound, and is often preceded by a snapping, clicking sound (so-called ejection sound); it has often a crescendo-decrescendo quality and ends before the second sound. In aortic stenosis, it is maximal in the third left and second right interspaces and is well heard over the suprasternal notch and the carotid arteries; it can be heard much lower, even at the apex. In subaortic stenosis (especially the muscular type), it is maximal over the left ventricular area. In pulmonary stenosis, the murmur is best heard over the second left intercostal space (pulmonary area), radiates moderately downwards, can be followed to the first left intercostal space, and often can be heard in the back (pulmonic areas).

The *murmur of semilunar valve insufficiency* is soft, high-pitched, blowing, occasionally musical, and (on auscultation) is in decrescendo. However, graphic tracings reveal that it may have a crescendo-decrescendo configuration and that it may be pandiastolic. In aortic insufficiency, the murmur is loudest in the third left interspace and can be followed along the left sternal border and toward the apex; it may be heard only at the apex. If the ascending aorta is dilated, the murmur is louder in the second right interspace and can be followed best along the right sternal border. In pulmonary insufficiency, the murmur is at times more rumbling; it is loudest over the second left interspace and can be followed downward and sometimes along an oblique line from the upper left to the lower right part of the sternum.

The murmur caused by a *ventricular septal defect (VSD)* is a long, harsh, pansystolic murmur. It is heard best in the third or fourth left intercostal space and can be followed toward the right precordium (right ventricular area). Exceptions are represented by the muscular type of VSD and by VSD associated with pulmonary hypertension.

The murmur caused by *patency of the ductus arteriosus* is a continuous murmur with accentuation in late-systole and early-diastole. It is heard best over the first and second left intercostal spaces. Exceptions occur in cases of complicated ductus, especially in infants, where the murmur may be only systolic, often with accentuation in late systole.

SHAPE AND PHASE OF MURMURS

Phonocardiography has revealed the shape and phase of murmurs, which had been surmised by means of auscultation. Unfortunately, certain shapes and phases that had been considered pathognomonic may be related to various structural or functional alternations, which will be discussed below.

Systolic Murmurs

An *early-systolic murmur in decrescendo* may result from mitral or tricuspid insufficiency, unimportant inflow tract changes, or ventricular septal defect (muscular type).

A *pansystolic murmur* may be caused by mitral or tricuspid insufficiency or ventricular septal defect.

A *late-systolic murmur in crescendo* usually indicates mitral insufficiency, but may be caused by patent ductus arteriosus (with pulmonary hypertension), ventricular aneurysm, adhesive pericarditis, muscular subaortic stenosis, or even pulmonary stenosis.

A *crescendo-decrescendo murmur* suggests aortic or pulmonary stenosis, flow murmur of the left or right outflow tract, mitral insufficiency (unusual), or ventricular septal defect (with pulmonary hypertension).

Diastolic Murmurs

An *early and mid-diastolic high frequency murmur in decrescendo* suggests aortic or pulmonary insufficiency (organic or relative).

An *early, mid- and late-diastolic (presystolic) rumble* indicates either mitral or tricuspid stenosis or inflow tract murmurs caused by a functional mechanism.

Double and Combined Murmurs

Double murmurs are murmurs which are present both in systole and diastole. However, they are separated by the heart sounds. They develop because of the existence of a double lesion of the same valve (insufficiency and stenosis). *Combined murmurs* are caused by stenosis of one valve and insufficiency of another or a similar lesion of two valves.

Continuous Murmurs

A *continuous murmur* usually results from a shunt, like patent ductus arteriosus, an AV fistula (systemic, pulmonary or coronary) or anastomotic vessels; however, it may be caused by either coarctation or an aneurysm of the aorta.

Chapter 14

Pitfalls of Auscultation

RAPID OR DISORDERED heart action, faintness of heart sounds or murmurs and certain limitation of the auditory system of man (Chapter 5) cause frequent errors of auscultation. Listed below are some of those most commonly encountered. Training of the observer, listening while watching sound on an oscilloscope, or recording a phonocardiogram, correct the error.

1. On account of rapid heart rate, systole and diastole may have about the same duration. Then the first and the second heart sound cannot be distinguished by the length of the phases that precede and follow them. This phenomenon was once called *embryocardia* because it is commonly observed as a normal phenomenon in the newborn. If there is one soft, blowing, high-pitched murmur that follows one of the heart sounds, it may be difficult to recognize whether it is systolic or diastolic.

2. Two acoustic phenomena indicating splitting of the first heart sound may be confused on auscultation. The first is the normal splitting of young people (components *a* and *b* are heard); the second is the slightly abnormal splitting of mature or elderly people (components *a* and *c* are heard) (Fig. 18).

3. Two phenomena in systole can be confused on auscultation.

The first is the early-systolic ejection sound, the second is the mid-systolic ejection click (Fig. 44).

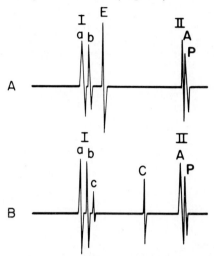

FIGURE 44. Possible auscultatory confusion between ejection sound (E) and systolic click (C).

4. Four acoustic phenomena in late-diastole (presystole) may be mistaken for each other on auscultation (Fig. 45) : a large and prolonged fourth sound (presystolic gallop), a crescendo presystolic murmur, a presystolic friction rub, and a physiologic, crescendo type of the first sound. A snapping and accentuated first heart sound is typical after the presystolic murmur of mitral stenosis but not after a functional presystolic rumble. The fourth sound is usually well separated from the following first sound but so is the presystolic rub, the presystolic murmur of tricuspid stenosis, and even the presystolic murmur of mitral stenosis if the patient has a grade 1 AV block.

5. Four acoustic phenomena in late systole or early diastole may be mistaken for each other on auscultation (Fig. 46) ; a late-systolic, high-pitched click followed by a normal second sound, a widely split second sound, a single second sound followed by an opening snap, and a single second sound followed by a loud third sound (ventricular gallop). Certain indirect data help for the differentiation. The splitting of the second sound

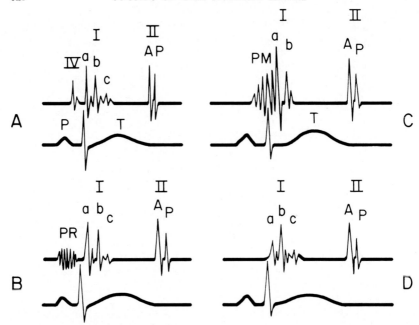

FIGURE 45. Possible auscultatory confusion of a large fourth sound (A) with a presystolic rub (B), a presystolic murmur (C) or a crescendo-type of the first heart sound (D).

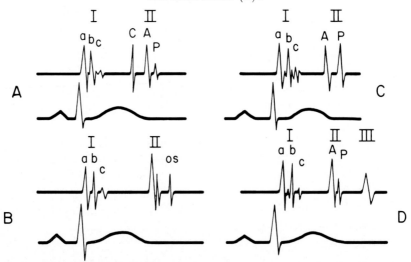

FIGURE 46. Possible auscultatory confusion between a late-systolic click (A), an early-diastolic opening snap (B), a widely split second sound (C), and a large third sound (D).

is best heard over the II-III left intercostal spaces and varies with respiration. The opening snap is best heard over the IV left intercostal space close to the sternum. The large third sound is duller than the others and is usually heard best over the apex. The systolic click is high-pitched and is usually heard over a wide area. However, a widely split second sound may be fixed (like in atrial septal defect or right bundle branch block), the third sound may be more high-pitched, and the opening snap may be heard over a wide area.

Part V

TECHNICAL ASPECTS OF PHONOCARDIOGRAPHY

Chapter 15

General Principles and Practical Aspects

MODERN PHONOCARDIOGRAPHY started its technical development with the invention of the amplifying triode by De Forest in 1906. However, amplifier units for audio work became commercially available only after 1920 in connection with the development of the radio.

Phonocardiography should be defined as *the graphic registration of the various bands of the precordial vibratory spectrum.* As such, phonocardiography should include the study of: (1) the infrasonic band; (2) the lower subliminal parts of the auditory band; (3) the audible components of the auditory band; and (4) the upper subliminal parts of the auditory band.

Given the physical dimensions and the dynamic range of the vibratory spectrum (a pressure or amplitude range of 1:1 million over 1,000 cycles), linear registration is impossible. The dynamic range of the ear is 120 db (10^{12} energy range), and the upper part of the vibratory spectrum of the heart is well within its range.

A *transducer* is basically a linear device, so that the electromotive force generated by this device is a direct function of pressure or displacement (Beranek). The dynamic range that can be recorded by such a system is unable to contain the spectrum in its totality while retaining a measure of clarity and detail for the vibrations in the high-frequency range.

It is evident that any attempt to register the high-frequency, low-energy components requires the attentuation of the low-frequency components. Two methods can be used.

1. An *equalizer* can be inserted in the circuit at a specific turnover frequency of the same but opposite slope; this would reduce the spectrum to a flat frequency characteristic by attentuating the low frequencies below such frequency, and boosting the frequencies above it. The converted spectrum can then be linearly amplified to any desired level. The final tracing, though physically modified, is supposed to reproduce all frequency components of the total spectrum. An equalizer was used in the Sanborn Stetho-Cardiette and in the Sanborn Twin-Beam recorder.

2. The frequency spectrum can be subdivided into adjoining bands through the use of *band-pass** or *high-pass*** *filters*. The frequency band passing through the filter is then amplified to the desired level for recording. Evidently the bands in question should cover the entire spectrum if complete scanning is desired. Therefore, several subsequent records should be taken for the various bands of the complex impulse.

The essential elements of a phonocardiograph include the transducer, the amplifier, the equalizer or filter, the recording system, and the transcription system (Fig. 47).

TRANDUCERS (MICROPHONES)

The microphone is the critical element of the phonocardiograph; it converts sound into electricity or, more exactly, it converts the energy contents of the vibratory spectrum into electric pulses of a certain voltage. An ideal microphone should have an electric output that is a faithful, undistorted image of the sound energy at the input. Sound energy is proportional to the product of frequency squared times amplitude squared. The amplitude of the vibrations is supposed to decrease in inverse proportion to the square of the frequency, i.e., with a slope of —12 db per octave.† Both linear and nonlinear distortions must be kept

---

*A band-pass filter was suggested by Luisada and Zalter in 1960 and was used by us for the construction of an experimental phonocardiograph. It is also used in our current equipment.

**High-pass RC filters were first used by European builders of phonocardiographs and have now great diffusion. They undoubtedly have the advantage of durability, low noise, and low cost.

†This point will be discussed in Part VII and was already discussed in Chap. 10.

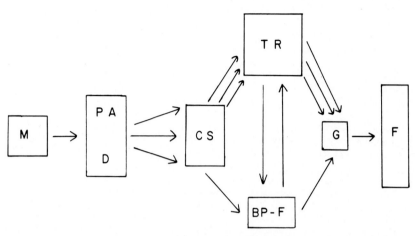

FIGURE 47. Scheme of a modern phonocardiograph. M = microphone; PA,D = preamplifier, differentiator; D,V,A = cables of displacement, velocity, and acceleration tracings; CS = connector switches; TR = tape recorder; BP-F = band pass filter; g = galvanometers; F = film.

low, and extraneous or interfering vibrations must be reduced to a minimum.

The microphone converts the vibratory motion of the chest wall, either directly or indirectly, into deflection of a diaphragm, coil, or ribbon.

In the *indirect method,* a closed air chamber is interposed so that the displacement is transformed into pressure, which then acts on the diaphragm. In the *direct method,* the diaphragm is brought into contact with the skin, either directly or through a connecting rod or probe *(contact microphone).* Perfect coupling has been attempted by juxtaposing the skin to a capacitor plate (Groom and Sihvonen).

Both the mode with which the deflection of the diaphragm is converted into electromotive force and the particular aspect of the oscillation that is transduced (displacement versus velocity or acceleration of a sinusoidal wave) determine the electric behavior of the microphone.

Transducers for Ultralow and Low-frequency Tracings

Transducers for ultralow- and low-frequency tracings include displacement, velocity, and acceleration transducers.

Displacement Transducers. For the purpose of apex car-
diography or other precordial tracings, the Sanborn No. 374
linear microphone can be used (Miller and White; Luisada,
1953; Dunn and Rahm, 1953; Luisada and Magri, 1952;
Benchimol *et al.,* 1961). The linear response is obtained by
the use of a crystal microphone, which is uniformly sensitive
to pressure changes from zero to several thousand hertz. It is
obvious in practice that such a microphone is limited in its response: (1) by the inability of the alternating current amplifier
(AC amplifier) to record extremely low-frequency vibrations
(0 to 2 hz) without some degree of distortion; (2) by the in-
adequacy of the galvanometer to record the extremely small
high-frequency vibrations; and (3) by the fact that the tre-
mendous magnitude of the ultralow-frequency vibrations (0 to
10 hz) makes it impossible to record the first and second sounds
and the murmurs with adequate amplification. Thus, the linear
system is inadequate for correctly recording extremely slow movements (0 to 1 hz) like those of respiration; it is adequate for
recording the pulses of ultralow frequency (1 to 5 hz correspond
to the apex beat, other chest wall pulsations, the epigastric beat,
and the hepatic, venous, or arterial pulses), though with a minor
degree of distortion; it is too comprehensive for the study of low-
frequency vibrations (1 to 30 hz); and it is definitely inadequate
for other purposes.*

The *kinetocardiogram* of the apex beat and other precordial
pulsations is recorded by a Statham PM5 transducer and a stiff
system of suspension (Eddleman *et al.,* 1953).

A Philips displacement meter and transducer with a frequency response of 0 to 70 hz was used by Schneider and Klun-
haar. Both record best the vibrations in the 0 to 30 hz range.

Velocity Transducers. A precordial velocity tracing may be
recorded by using a Sanborn electromanometer with a differential
circuit (Johnson and Overy).

Acceleration Transducers. A precordial acceleration tracing
can be obtained by using a piezoelectric transducer (Statham

---

*The Hewlett-Packard Co. has introduced in its latest equipment a new contact
microphone that can be used for both apex cardiogram and heart sounds,
recording through two different amplifiers and filters.

Transducers, Inc.; Consolidated Electrodynamics) or an electromagnetic transducer (F & G Sound, Chicago; Shure Bros., No. 61CP, Evanston, Illinois). The electromagnetic device has the advantage that it can be connected to the amplifier of a conventional electrocardiograph. Vibrations in the 5 to 30 hz range are best sensed by this device.

Simultaneous Records of Precordial Acceleration, Velocity, and Displacement. In our laboratory, a single and double differentiation system is used in order to obtain simultaneous records of precordial displacement, velocity, and acceleration. This technique permits a good visualization of the low, medium and high frequency components of the precordial pulsation. The simultaneous registration of these aspects of the pulsation combines the advantages of the three single methods.

Well-defined physical characteristics of any system and exact data on its frequency response are necessary for accurate and meaningful registration because most transducers operate with an optimum performance in a given frequency range.

Transducers for Sound Tracings

The choice of a transducer for reproducing audible vibrations is a difficult problem.

Basically, microphones can sense either *displacement* (crystal and capacitor microphones), *velocity* (dynamic and magnetic transducers), or *acceleration* (piezoelectric and electromagnetic transducers).

In both the crystal and the capacitor microphones, the electromotive force (EMF), generated at any given moment, is directly proportional to the deflection of the diaphragm, which in turn is a function of the pressure changes applied at the input. The design of both microphones is such as to ensure that the ratio between the final deflection and the pressure applied is independent of frequency (Dunn and Rahm, 1952). Both are *displacement microphones.**

Examples of the *crystal microphone* used in phonocardiography are the Sanborn stethoscopic and logarithmic microphones used in conjunction with the old Stetho-Cardiette, the Cambridge

---

*In industry, piezoelectric transducers are widely used as accelerometers.

(U.S.A.) microphone, and the Peiker microphone used in conjunction with the Electronics for Medicine recorder. In all the above, there is an indirect transmission, the air of a chest piece acting on the diaphragm. Another type of crystal microphone, however, uses a direct contact with the skin (contact microphone). An example of this type is the Maico 48-A-10, also employed by Sanborn.

Examples of the *capacitor or condenser microphone* are the Altec-Lansing microphones, which are widely used in radio and television transmission. The 21-D microphone was used in our experimental phonocardiograph.

In the *dynamic microphone,* the diaphragm is brought into motion by the varying pressure within the closed chamber; however, the diaphragm in this case carries a conductor (or coil) positioned in a constant magnetic field. The EMF generated is proportional to the rate of displacement (velocity), which in turn is proportional to the product of the amplitude squared times the frequency. Thus the tracing is a record of the velocity aspect of the vibrations, i.e., of the first derivative of the displacement of the vibrating surface. An example of the dynamic microphone is the model 62-1500-C10 used by the Sanborn Company in both the Twin-Beam (1950) and the 564 system (1960). In the latter, a transformer is interposed between microphone and amplifier to match the high impedance of the amplifier. The microphone-transformer has a great sensitivity for medium- and high-frequency vibrations but has a low response in the range of the 20 to 40 hz frequencies (low subliminal band).

Another type of velocity transducer is the *magnetic type.* An example of this is the SP-5S (Shure Bros.), which records by direct contact with the skin.

None of the currently used types has an absolute advantage or superiority; their merits are only relative and are partly the result of the peculiarity of the phenomenon under study. For a vibratory spectrum sloping in amplitude at 12 to 15 db per octave, the high-frequency vibrations are at a great disadvantage because of their extremely small amplitude. The use of displacement microphone, irrespective of its performance characteristics, favors the predominance of low-frequency elements in the tracing, even though the final picture is an exact replica of the various amplitudes as they appear at the surface of the chest wall.

A velocity microphone, on the other hand, tends to emphasize higher frequency elements (Kountz et al., 1940; Smith, J. R. et al., 1941; Johnston and Overy).

Other factors should be considered in the selection of a microphone, i.e., the nature of the sound field, the dynamic range, and the frequency range.

Nature of the Sound Field: Considering the intensity level of the vibratory phenomenon, free-field transmission is ruled out for the present, and transmission can be either direct or indirect. In the *direct method,* either a double-walled suction funnel surrounding the button or a ring of sponge rubber in a grooved casing is applied on the chest. In the *indirect method,* the shape, volume, and dimensions of the closed chamber are critical factors because the cavity resonance may distort the response of the microphone at the resonant frequencies (Dunn and Rahm, 1953). However, if the volume of the bell is kept large enough (around 10 cubic centimeters) with a ratio of diameter to height of 3:1, the response characteristics remain linear up to the resonance point, well above the upper frequency range of the sound spectrum (Rappaport and Sprague, 1941).

Dynamic Range. The microphone should be capable of transducing with equal fidelity the components that are at the two extreme ends of the spectrum (Rodbard et al., 1955, Dunn, 1957). At the upper frequency range of the spectrum the amplitude may be as low as 0.01 to 0.001 dyne per square centimeter and the microphone will be able to transduce such a weak impulse only through a high-sensitivity and low-noise level.*

The limiting factor is the thermal noise voltage. The noise can be expressed in terms of the equivalent sound pressure, theoretically generated in an ideally silent microphone. A signal, to be usefully transduced, should be at least from 20 to 30 db above the level of self-noise in order to stand clearly above the base line.

The self-noise generated by a microphone over a band of

---

*The *sensitivity of a microphone* can be defined as the amount of output voltage for a given vibratory amplitude or energy input.

three decades (10 to 10,000 hz) can be equated to a sound pressure level of 10 to 20 db above the threshold pressure of the human ear (0.0002 dyne per square centimeter). Since the magnitude of the signal should be at least 20 db above the noise level, the threshold pressure that such a coil microphone can efficiently transduce is 40 db higher than the threshold pressure of the human ear.

The sensitivity of the mircophone is linear over a wide band, whereas the sensitivity of the ear varies as a function of frequency. Nevertheless, in the high-frequency range, the ear is just as sensitive as, or more so than, a well-designed coil microphone.

Frequency Range. The frequency response of most microphones is linear over the major part of the spectrum of the human ear (Dunn and Rahm, 1953; Miller and White). A calibration curve of the microphone indicates the open-circuit voltage that is produced as a function of the frequency for a constant sound pressure (Dunn and Rahm, 1953A; Miller and White, McGregor *et al.*). The constant sound pressure,* generally used in conjunction with calibration, is 1 dyne per square centimeter.

Our New Microphone

Our current set-up has been built by the General Electric Company of Schenectady, New York. The microphone is a *General Radio* 1560 P-5 with a frequency response of ± 3 db re IV/μ bar from 10 to 1,000 hz with a sensitivity of at least—60 db re IV/μ bar. It is a piezoelectric transducer recording displacement and it is based on air transmission. Its characteristics are as follows:

cavity diameter	20 mm
cavity depth	8 mm
contact surface loading	1.8 gm/cm
total assembled weight	70 gm
material	aluminum

The microphone is provided of a *General Radio Acoustic Calibrator Unit.* Calibration of displacement, first stage (ve-

---

*The use of a *constant sound pressure* for calibration has been expedient in the past. However, the need for calibration in terms of the energy content of vibrations has become apparent.

locity), and second stage (acceleration) differentiation is obtained through this unit.

The calibration of the first stage shows a gain slope of 20 db/decade without filtration, yielding a voltage output equivalent to the first differentiation of displacement. However, to achieve a voltage gain of 40 db/decade, equivalent to the second differentiation of displacement, it was necessary to band reject more than 3,000 hz.

Even though the signal-to-noise ratio for double differentiation is adequate for data processing, it is greatly enhanced when a narrow band pass filter is utilized.

The Self Noise of the Differentiator is as Follows:

Second Differentiation—Acceleration $= 9 \times 10^{-9}$ in/sec (f)

First Differentiation—Velocity $\quad = 1.5 \times 10^{-8}$ g (f)

f = frequency

The range of amplification for both signal and noise can be as much as 80 db between an input at 10 hz and output at 1000 hz.

EQUALIZERS

Basically, an equalizer is a device for altering the frequency characteristics of a recording system (Pender, Terman).

An equalizer is a variable-loss device controlled by the applied frequencies, which in turn vary the gain of the system in a given frequency range. When several frequencies are simultaneously applied to the input of an equalizer, their amplitude relative to each other is altered at the output. If the equalizer has inverse frequency characteristics to those of the vibratory spectrum, the spectrum is transformed to flat frequency characteristics. In so doing, the overall signal level will be lowered (insertion loss). The signal may then be returned to its original level by amplification.

Phase Distortion. This phenomenon assumes a great importance in the ultralow- and low-frequency region of the spectrum (1 to 40 hz) where the shape and configuration of the waves are of diagnostic significance. In the medium high-frequency region (above 100 hz), a certain amount of phase distortion can be tolerated without affecting the final configuration of the sound under study. A delay below 20 msec. at 100 hz in relation to the delay at 1,000 hz is tolerable from a graphic point of view but is not acceptable for accurate scientific investigations.

The equalizers are composed of elements consisting of a resistor, inductor, and capacitor, connected according to a definite scheme and specific types. These elements offer an obstacle to the passage of certain frequencies and thus control the frequency rsponse of the system.

AMPLIFIERS

An amplifier is a device whose main function is to magnify and faithfully reproduce the essential features of an electric wave of small energy applied to the input. The output represents a greater amount of energy because the amplifier draws power from a source other than the signal.

Amplifiers belong to different classes. When the voltages at input and output have a linear relation, the amplifier is designated as a *Class A amplifier*. Partial operation of the amplifier in the nonlinear region during a fraction of the cycle results in an output wave that does not exactly reproduce the signal. Such an amplifier shows the wave and is generally designated as *Class AB, B, or C* depending upon the degree of nonlinearity.

As the amplification derived from a single stage of amplification may be insufficient, one resorts to connection of two or more stages (multistage or cascade amplifier) connected by a coupling network. The type of coupling determines the range of frequencies over which it operates.

Ideally, an amplifier is supposed to produce at the output a wave form that duplicates exactly that received at the input except in magnitude. However, even minor imperfections cause some difference between the shape of the wave at the input and output. Such a deviation from the ideal, called *frequency distortion,* limits the range of frequencies that can be satisfactorily handled.

On the other hand, an amplifier that distorts the shape of the frequency components (this may occur when operating in the nonlinear region of the tube characteristics) is responsible for nonlinear or amplitude distortion. Finally, if the amplifier fails to preserve the time relationship among the various components, the output wave is said to suffer from *phase distortion.*

Amplification or gain. The gain can be expressed as the *ratio of the voltage at the output to that at the input.* However, since the signal is usually a complex wave, the gain for the various frequency components may not be the same. A more accurate picture of the gain can be obtained from the curve of frequency response, which is *a plot of the voltage gain versus frequency on a logarithmic scale.* Gain may then be expressed either in absolute numbers or in decibels above the original input level of 0 db.

Amplifier Coupling. The type of coupling between two stages of an amplifier determines to a large extent the characteristics of its frequency response. When it is desired to transmit steady direct current (DC) potentials (or variations of less than 1 hz), direct coupling must be resorted to; this type is called a direct current amplifier *(DC amplifier)* and is used for the study of ultra-low or low-frequency pulsations. For frequencies above 1 hz, and where the DC component of the complex wave need not be transmitted or amplified, an alternating current amplifier *(AC amplifier)* is the unit of choice.

Noise. Electric noise is the major limiting factor in the performance of a transducer-amplifier system. The noise level generated by such a system sets the minimal limit of intensity of a signal because greater amplification amplifies both the noise and the signal so that the separation between the signal and the artifacts is not increased. This means that the possibility of reading a signal is a function of the *signal-to-noise ratio* or, in different terms, of a narrow base line (Groom). Since the fluctuations of noise are random, their frequencies are evenly distributed over a wide band of the frequency spectrum. As a result, the noise level at the output becomes a function of the band-width being recorded. Limiting the band-width to the frequency spectrum of the signal under study improves the resolution of the amplifier by increasing the signal-to-noise ratio at the output. This is performed best by means of a band-pass filter (Luisada and Zalter, 1960).

In our present set up, Sanborn 350-2700c amplifiers are used. In general, the DC input gives sufficient amplification but the AC input can also be used in case of extremely small signals.

FILTERS

Filters used in phonocardiography are either acoustic or electric; the latter includes low-pass and band-pass filters.

Acoustic filters. Acoustic filters cannot be considered ideal because the degree and extent of attenuation is a function of several factors, which cannot always be accurately controlled. Acoustic filters were used in the Sanborn Stetho-Cardiette.

Electric filters. An electric filter is a network whose function is to pass a given band of frequencies without appreciable attenuation and to attenuate all others. The frequency that marks the junction of a pass band with an attenuation band is known as the *cutoff frequency,* and the rate at which frequencies outside the pass band are attenuated is determined by the *slope.* From the standpoint of frequency characteristics, the filters are of three types: (1) low-pass filters, (2) high-pass filters, and (3) band-pass filters. In the *low-pass filters,* all frequencies above cutoff frequency are attenuated at a specified slope; in the *high-pass filters,* those frequencies below a cutoff frequency are attenuated; a *band-pass filter* allows a specified range of frequencies through the combination of high- and low-pass filters.

IC (Inductance-capacitance) Filters. IC filters have been used with good results. They have certain drawbacks that can prove critical, however, because the inductance necessary to handle the low frequencies can be large, and IC filters tend to pick up interference unless a careful screening is obtained. A second undesirable feature is the considerable variation of phase with frequency within the pass band. Introduction of resonant harmonics often results.

RC (Resistance-capacitance) Filters. RC filters are particularly suited for biologic work involving vibration studies and in conjunction with any low-frequency phenomenon involving selective amplification. Filters, either high or low, can be constructed by coupling two or more RC units in series. Since the rate of attenuation of each unit is 6 db per octave, the net rate of attenuation is a function of the number of units so coupled. For example, four RC units would produce an attenuation rate of 24 db per octave. The cutoff frequency of such a high-pass filter does not correspond to the point at which the slope of the filter curve asymptotically intersects the 0 db line; instead, it has been shifted to the left (toward the lower frequencies) because, by definition, the cutoff frequency is that frequency at which the output of the filter is 3 db down (50 per cent) from the output at the pass band. This can be corrected by the introduction of a peaking circuit* to sharpen the corner of the slope (i.e., to increase the slope in the corner area). The performance of such a filter is far superior to that of an average filter because of the increased gain near the corner frequency. Therefore, it is possible to reduce and practically eliminate the curved upper critical portion of the RC-filtered curve at the expense of an increased complexity of the system.

The insertion of a high-pass filter involves certain problems of particular importance in phonocardiography (Maass and Weber; Holldack and Wolf). Maass and Weber suggested the adoption of a point of reference (500 hz), the transmission of which can be regarded as 100 per cent of input (its attenuation would then be 0 db). The point of 10 per cent transmission (90 per cent down or 20 db attenuation) can be regarded as the rated frequency of a given filter. Below the rated frequency, the slope of the filter (which is logarithmic) determines the rate of attenuation in decibels per octave. The frequency of maximal amplitude *(normal frequency)*** does not correspond to the rated frequency and is somewhat above it.

By grossly spacing the rated frequency at octave intervals of 35, 70, 140, 250, and 500 hz† and keeping the slope constant at 24 db per octave (except for the lowest frequencies of 35 and 70 hz, which have a slope of 7.5 db per octave and 18 db per octave, respectively), the spectrum was divided by Maass and Weber into adjacent and partly overlapping bands, which were then amplified with a ratio of 1:4 per octave. This ratio is supposed to compensate for the decreasing magnitude that occurs with increasing frequency. Thus, through the exclusive use of high-pass filters, strategically placed at octave intervals, the

*Peaking can be obtained by using a capacitor-inductor tuned circuit.

**The nominal frequency corresponds to a point on the filter curve whose slope is equal but opposite in sign to the slope of the vibratory spectrum.

†Zalter and I (1960) have employed a similar spacing at 50, 100, 200, 400 and 800 hz.

spectrum is split into bands suitable for amplification and recording.

In a modification of the Sanborn equipment used in our
laboratory, different slopes were adopted for the different filters,
based on the need of a wider range for lower frequencies.*

Band-pass Filters. A band-pass filter is made of a high-pass
and low-pass filter connected in series. Such a filter incorporates
the characteristics of both the high- and the low-pass sections.
Band-pass filters were studied by several authors (Frederick and
Dodge; Mannheimer; Zalter *et al.;* Luisada and Zalter, 1960).
Williams and Dodge used a system incorporating a band-pass
filter as an auscultatory wave analyzer. However, the clinical use
of such a system for auscultatory analysis cannot be justified because of the addition of a physiologic system to a physical system.

In the operation of a band-pass filter, the interaction of the
peaking circuits of both the high and low cutoff frequencies
should be taken into consideration. For a pass band of one octave,
however, it should be possible to obtain a band with 0 db in
the center and a 3 db loss at the nominal cutoff frequency. To
increase the peaking of the circuit, Jacono and Friedland, Faber
and Burton, and Shah *et al* (1963A), have used a Krohn-Hite
band-pass filter by applying both the high-pass and the low-pass
filters at the same point (100 to 100, 200 to 200, etc).

Our present band pass filter is a Krohn-Hite 3342 with the
following characteristics:

frequency range	0.001 to 99.9 Khz
passband gain	1 or 10 (voltage)
band-pass attenuation slope	48 db/octave
maximal attenuation	80 db

The type of operation selected was that described by Butterworth. By setting the two cutoff frequencies at the same figure,
the insertion loss if 6 db and the —3 db cutoff frequencies occur
at 0.9 and 1.12 times the midband frequency. This unit is essentially made of two separate filters, employed for low-pass and
high-pass rejection. They can be also employed in series. In such
a case, the slope of the filter will be 96 db/octave.

---

*Similar filters were used by Yoshimura.

RECORDING SYSTEMS

The recording device can be either a cathode-ray tube or a galvanometer.

Cathode-ray Tube. The cathode-ray tube is the most accurate and sensitive recording device. Unlike other means of recording, it is free from the effect of inertia and hence its frequency response is unlimited. In conjunction with a blue fluorescence of high actinic value, it is suitable for photography. If connected with a system recording on bromide paper, however, the cathode-ray tube is less than ideal because, when high-frequency vibrations are being inscribed, the faster the spot moves, the fainter the trace becomes. The use of an electronic switch for multiple recording further detracts from the clarity and resolution of the record in the high-frequency range. The use of the more expensive double-beam of multiple-beam tubes with separate gun assemblies could obviate this drawback.

The *oscilloscope** has been used in recent years in a different way:** If the R wave of the electrocardiogram is used to trigger the onset of sweep of one or more beams, one can constantly visualize either both heart sounds (slow-sweep speed), or one of them (medium-sweep speed), or part of one of them (high-sweep speed), as well as fractions of systole or diastole. A *camera†* can then be used to photograph the rapidly moving spot on the screen of the oscilloscope. High-speed phonocardiography is based on this arrangement (Caniggia and Bertelli‡; Dunn and Rahm, 1953; Sterz; Faber and Burton; and Shah *et al.*, 1963A). It is undoubtedly the best method for studying the speed of transmission of the sound waves over the chest wall or the number of harmonics of the fundamental sound wave.** Sweeps of from 600 to over 1,000 mm per second have been used.

---

*The first oscilloscope, applied to cardiovascular studies by Rosa (1939), was called a *cardioscope.*

**The Dual-beam Dumont oscilloscope No. 411 is one of the oscilloscopes that can be used for this purpose.

†A Polaroid Land camera (Model 95) has been used by us, together with a blue filter in front of the P-7 screen of the oscilloscope.

‡The method of Caniggia records the output of a single microphone through several channels with various filters. It is obvious that channels with high filtration will have too small waves unless separate amplification is used.

GALVANOMETERS

Recording oscillographs incorporating moving-coil galvanometers or their modifications are commonly used in conjunction with amplifying circuits for recording either low- or high-frequency vibrations.

String Galvanometer. The string galvanometer, perfected to a high degree of sensitivity and frequency response prior to the advent of modern electronics, has now only a limited use in phonocardiography.

Moving-coil Galvanometer. The moving-coil galvanometer (D'Arsonval) is commonly used in phonocardiography. The moving element consists of a coil of fine wire suspended between taut suspension strips and mounted in a strong magnetic field. Current is conducted to the coil through one strip and out through the other, causing the coil to turn and twist the strips. A mirror is mounted on the coil. Such an arrangement can be compared to an elastic system with an instantaneous deflection, which is at all times proportional to the forces acting upon it.

The moving-coil galvanometer is less accurate than the cathode-ray tube in regard to flat frequency response and phase relationship but, when properly chosen to cover the desired range of frequencies and damped accordingly, it is accurate enough for most applications. By using a multielement magnet block, a large number of galvanometers can be enclosed in a small space for multiple recording.

All galvanometers have definite limitations in sensitivity and frequency. In the selection of a galvanometer for a specific application, it is necessary to weigh the relative importance of each of the four main characteristics: frequency response, sensitivity, phase angle, and damping. A compromise between the various characteristics is obviously necessary.

Frequency Response. In order to perform over a wide frequency range, yet be relatively flat, most galvanometers are so designed that, when damped to 64.5 per cent of critical damping, they have a flat response with ±5 per cent of the final response up to 60 per cent of their undamped natural frequency. Fluid-damped galvanometers have a frequency response of from 30 to 50 per cent of their undamped natural frequency.

Current Sensitivity. Maximum current sensitivity is always associated with maximum resistance and minimum natural frequency. If a higher frequency is desired, it must be remembered that a lower sensitivity is a necessary result. Therefore, a more powerful amplifier will be needed.

Damping: The two methods of damping that are normally used are (1) the electromagnetic damping for galvanometers having a low natural frequency (usually less than 500 hz) and (2) the fluid damping for galvanometers having a high natural frequency. When using galvanometers that require electromagnetic damping, it is important that the correct input impedance be used to ensure the specific flat frequency response. In fluid-damped galvanometers, the input impedance will have little effect on the frequency response.

TRANSCRIPTION SYSTEMS

The transcription of the phonocardiogram is made in one of the following ways:

1. By projecting on photographic bromide film the light beam of a galvanometer.
2. By projecting on photographic bromide film the light beam of a cathode-ray tube.
3. By one of the various methods of direct writing or rapid writing phonocardiography.
   (a) The Schwarzer Company and the Hellige Company (both of Germany) have succeeded in obtaining a curve envelope for the higher frequencies.* In such apparatus, duration, amplitude, and variations in amplitude of the vibrations are recorded but frequency analysis is not possible. The transcription is obtained by a heated stylus moving on a specially prepared paper.
   (b) The Elema Company (of Sweden) has used an ink jet delivered by a capillary tube not touching the paper, thus avoiding excessive inertia of the system and giving a fair reproduction of medium high-frequency vibrations (probably up to 300 to 400 hz).

---

*Rushmer *et al.* described the *sonvelogram.* This is obtained by half-wave rectification and electric integration and gives a tracing that corresponds to the intensity envelope of sound in its entirety.

(c) Several companies, including the Sanborn Company and Electronics for Medicine, have suggested a rapid method of automatic development that allows inspection of the tracing within a few seconds.

The first method undoubtedly gives a somewhat distorted picture of the tracing. The second method is still inadequate for the transcription of the highest frequencies. Moreover, further photographic reproductions of the tracing (for publication or duplication) is less than excellent. The third method is as good as the phonocardiographic system to which it is added but, again, the visual quality of the tracing is definitely less good than with the customary photographic system.

In our present system, the light beams of the various galvanometers are projected onto a special high speed photographic paper (Dataflash DP 1, from ECE). The tracings are brought out by exposure to ambient ultra-violet light and can either be fixed by a chemical process or protected from ultraviolet light.

In my opinion, the photographic system is still the best. Immediate study of the tracing can be obtained through use of an oscilloscope. Photographic processing of the film can be done by a technician, nurse, or an aide in the doctor's office or in the hospital. The loss of a few minutes is irrelevant because phonocardiography cannot be classified among the emergency procedures.

The recording film speed should be selected in view of the best identification of the vibrations of the phonocardiogram. It is obvious that a high recording speed will tend to spread (and thus seemingly flatten) the various waves. Thus, any high speed of recording will require a greater amplitude of the transcribed signal to compensate for the flattening effect.

A speed of 25 mm per second is used by several authors, either in order not to distort the simultaneously recorded electrocardiogram* or for the sake of economy. It is definitely inadequate. A speed of 50 mm per second is useful for a gross

---

*If the physician is interested in preserving the conventional picture of the electrocardiogram, the amplitude of this should be increased in proportion (2 cm per millivolt for a speed of 50 mm per second, 4 cm per millivolt for a speed of 100 mm per second, etc.).

evaluation of the body of a murmur; it is still inadequate for an accurate study of the tracing. A speed of 100 mm per second is currently used in our laboratory. Speeds of 200, 400 or 1,600 mm per second can be used for timing or analysis of high-frequency vibrations but are unnecessary in routine work. Higher speeds can be obtained by photographing the screen of an oscilloscope or with special equipment like the one in use in our laboratory.

VARIOUS PHONOCARDIOGRAPHS

A comparison and critical analysis of various existing systems was made by Zalter and Luisada (1954A).

An experimental phonocardiograph, based on the Altec-Lansing microphone and amplifiers, a Krohn-Hite band-pass filter, and British Electronics for Medicine galvanometers and camera, was built by Zalter and Luisada (1960). This apparatus gave an excellent transcription of high-frequency vibrations (Luisada and Di Bartolo).

In recent years, Bernstein and Luisada have modified the standard Sanborn equipment so that the following characteristics were incorporated.

1. Use of a dynamic microphone with transformer.
2. Use of high-pass filters with these characteristics:
   (a) Position 0 with no filtration, to be connected to a DC amplifier.
   (b) Position 50 with a slope of —6 db per octave.*
   (c) Position 100 with a slope of —12 db per octave.
   (d) Position 200 with a slope of —24 db per octave.
   (e) Position 400 with a slope of —24 db per octave.
   (f) Position 600 with a slope of —30 db per octave.**
3. Use of a second stage of amplification for the high frequencies so that the total power amplification reaches 120 db.
4. No automatic compensation for the decrement in amplitude of the high-frequency vibrations; use of a linear

---

*Some authors insist in designating the 50 hz point, i.e., that point at which the amplification has dropped approximately 50 per cent (3 db). The value that Maass and Weber would assign to our No. 50 filter would then be No. 7.

**Only a half octave separates the 400 from the 600 cps filter.

gain control, adjusted by the operator to obtain the optimal degree of amplification.

5. Use of either an electric or a sound calibrator.
6. Use of an oscilloscope for monitoring the tracing before and during the recording.

Calibrated Phonocardiography

Calibrated phonocardiography is based on the absolute linearity of the various components of a system. It was described by Mannheimer and was revived by Zalter and myself (1960). In our experimental apparatus, amplification was measured in decibels and similar tracings could be taken with identical amplification for the same frequency band. The problems of calibration are discussed in Chapter 17. Our present setup (see below) is based on a calibrated system.

Frequency Analysis

At present, three methods can be used for the study of selected bands of frequencies:

1. High-pass or band-pass filters can be used for recording simultaneous (multichannel phono) or subsequent (single-channel phono) tracings of heart sounds and murmurs in various adjoining octave bands and for comparison of the tracings. This is the most commonly used method and was pioneered by Mannheimer.

2. A variable band-pass filter can be used, and setting of both high- and low-pass filters at the same figures allows for subsequent records in that extremely narrow band that is allowed to pass in such technical conditions. This method was advocated by Jacono and Friedland in our laboratory and was used by Faber and Burton, and Shah et al. (1963). It is used in our present setup.

3. A *Spectrum analyzer,* as advocated by McKusick et al. (1954), Blume, Oberhoffer, and Ebina et al., can also be used.

McKusick's equipment is based on a device originally developed by Fletcher for the study of speech frequencies and intensities. It records a few heart cycles on a tape, rapidly scans these cycles by means of a variable filter, and then records on the final graph certain lines that indicate frequencies (ordinate) versus time (abscissa) plus their magnitude (blackness). It is unfortunate that so far technical reasons have prevented a better resolution of the final tracing, its spreading on a film having a higher speed, and its simultaneous recording with several other manifestations of cardiodynamics (conventional phonocardiogram, ECG, and pulse tracing).

OUR PRESENT EQUIPMENT

In 1969, we developed a new system for both experimental and clinical phonocardiography in collaboration with the R and D Section of the General Electric Company of Schenectady, N. Y. and with the aid of a grant of the F. Rippel Foundation of Newark, N. Y.

The new phonocardiograph is based on the following components: (Fig. 48A) (1) An air-coupled acoustic sensing unit (General Dynamics microphone) with a flat frequency response from 10 to 1000 hz and a sensitivity of at least —60 db. This is provided with either a suction system or a heavy rubber ring for skin application, and is routinely calibrated by means of a specially constructed device. Connected with this microphone are a pre-amplifier and single and double differentiation circuits made by the General Electric Company. Thus, signals corresponding to *displacement, velocity,* and *acceleration* are recorded. (2) A Krohn-Hite band-pass filter with a —48 db/octave attenuation slope. (3) A 60 db gain amplifier with a frequency range from 0 to 75 Khz. (4) A C.E.C. multi-speed magnetic tape recorder with 7 tracks. (5) An 8-channel Sanborn oscilloscope. (6) Seven C.E.C. galvanometers having a frequency response of 0 to 3000 hz. (7) A direct print-out light beam oscillograph with 17.5 cm. paper.

This equipment represents an electronic system for storage and display of signals. Connected with a multichannel Sanborn system for recording electrocardiograms, pressure tracings, flow tracings, and their derivatives, it lends itself to multiple experimental and clinical studies.

Another combination has been developed in our clinical laboratory. The above microphone and differentiator were con-

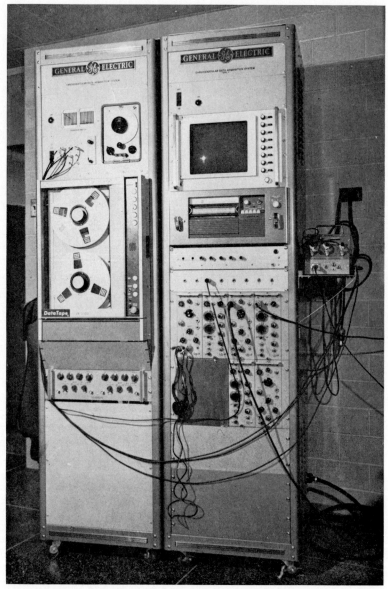

FIGURE 48. Our new phonocardiograph with tape recorder. (A) Model for
experimental studies. (B) Clinical model.

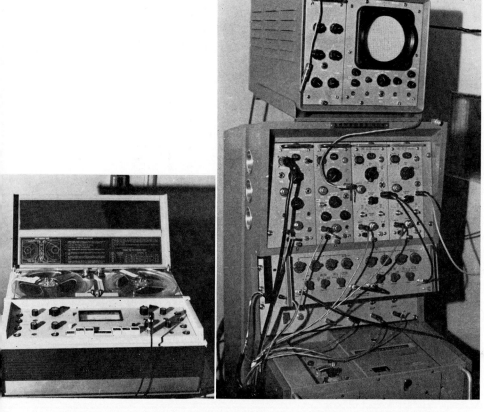

nected to: (a) a Krohn-Hite band pass filter with a —48 db/octave slope; (b) a series of Sanborn amplifiers with linear characteristics; (c) a series of high frequency Sanborn galvanometers; and (d) a Sanborn 4 track Tape Recorder (Fig. 48B). The same information is obtained as in the above device for experimental studies.

Chapter 16

Tape Recording. Computer Analysis

TAPE RECORDERS

TAPE RECORDERS are used to record heart sounds for subsequent review or analysis.

The operation of a tape recorder is basically that of magnetically coding an electric signal onto the thin oxide coating of a flexible tape. These signals can then be decoded and analysed at a later date.

Information can be stored on the tape as either amplitude-modulated (AM) or frequency modulated (FM) signals. The accuracy with which these signals can be recorded and reproduced depends on several factors: (1) the quality of the amplifiers that impress and retrieve the signals from the magnetic heads; (2) the quality of the tape; and (3) the speed with which the tape passes over the heads.

In general, the greater the speed, the greater the range of frequencies that the recorder will be capable of transcribing.

Because of physical limitations of the tape itself, the maximum dynamic range of most tape recorders is about 48 db. This means that the maximum intensity signal that can be recorded without distortion is 48 db above noise level.

Besides recording data, the tape recorder offers some interesting analysis features. Information recorded at one speed can

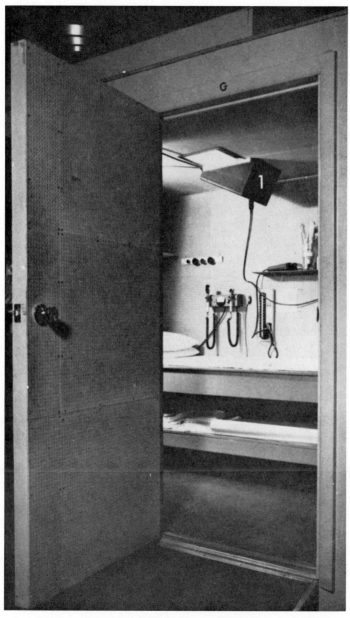

FIGURE 49. Sound proof chamber.

be played back at another speed for analysis. An unfiltered record can be passed through a filter before recording. Tapes may be formed into loops for repeated analysis. Information can even be played back backwards.

Recorded tape must be protected from stray magnetic fields like those emitted by x-ray machines, and the tape will lose its fidelity after many passes over the heads of the recorder.

Because of the relatively narrow dynamic range of the tape, signals may have to be broken up into several bands of frequencies by means of filters, and recorded on two or more channels, each with its own degree of amplification.

COMPUTER ANALYSIS

The role of the computer in analyzing heart sounds and murmurs is one of relieving the physician of making tedious and lengthy numerical comparisons.

The data concerning sounds and murmurs are changed into a form that can be recognized by the computers, such as a voltage or a digit. These data are then compared with normal values, which have been previously stored within the machine.

The combination of data points that fall outside the normal range is compared to the data of known disease entities, and the machine indicates the abnormal data and their most likely physical cause.

The main problem is that of recognizing normal values from a large enough population sample so that these can be fed to the machine as reference material.

Chapter 17

Calibration

CALIBRATION of sound vibrations is a technical problem, the importance of which is universally recognized.

Calibration is not currently employed for the following reasons:

1. The extremely different amplitude of the sound vibrations of the heart in the various frequency bands makes it impossible to use a single type of calibration signal.

2. The fact that vibrations of different frequencies are recorded in succession through different bands complicates the problem because the frequency of the calibrating signal should be similar to that of the recorded signal.

3. Between the source of the vibrations and the recorded signal are interposed: (a) the heart and vessels; (b) the extracardiac tissues; (c) the chest wall; (d) the microphone (and, except for contact microphones, the air interposed between the chest wall and the microphone); (e) the amplifier and filters; (f) the galvanometer or cathode-ray tube, and (g) the transcribing system.

It is obvious that two main sets of variables are involved, i.e., a set of anatomic and physiologic variables (a to c) and a set of technical variables (d to g).

Following the example of electrocardiography, the practitioner might try to calibrate initially the amplitude of a given signal, then increase or decrease the magnitude of the cardiac sounds until the calibration signal gives an electric pulse that is equivalent to the standard accepted degree of amplification; at this time they would take the record. This trend should be discouraged. Should this method be adopted, some of the tracings would present excessively large vibrations (exceeding the width of the recording film) whereas others would show only tiny vibrations, completely unsuitable for observation and study, or none at all.

Therefore, a second method should be used: the degree of amplification should be adjusted until the vibrations have the best amplitude for study (2 to 5 cm); then one would calibrate by means of a standard signal in order to establish the degree of amplification that had been used. The calibration signal should not be affected by the filters and should have a wide range of amplitude.

CALIBRATION OF MICROPHONES

Laboratory microphones are usually calibrated in terms of their open-circuit voltage for a given sound pressure in a free field (Beranek).

For phonocardiographic use, the *open-circuit pressure response* is suitable for calibration because it simulates the condition under which the microphone is used (Mannheimer, 1940; Dunn and Rahm, 1953A). The results are expressed in terms of open-circuit voltage for a constant sound pressure uniformly distributed over the diaphragm. For a reference voltage of 1 volt and a reference pressure of 1 dyne per square centimeter, the response in decibels is 20 log e/p, where e is the open-circuit voltage and p is the pressure at the diaphragm. For a microphone whose output level is —55 db, the voltage generated is 55 db below the reference level of 0 db (1 volt-dyne per square centimeter). Obviously, the smaller the number of decibels, the higher the output level and the more sensitive this is.[*] Once the sensitivity curve of a microphone is known, there is no need for frequent checking: this curve will persist unchanged unless the microphone is damaged, a fact that is easily revealed by gross artifacts and by an increase of noise during the silent phases of cardiodynamics.

Even though constant sound pressure has been used for calibration in the past, the need for calibration in terms of the energy output of vibrations is now deeply felt. This would require a different mode of evaluation of the output of microphones.

A *sound calibrator* was devised by Olson and Massa and modified by Stodel and by Dunn and Rahm (1953), who based their devices on the comparison of two juxtaposed cathode-ray beams. A second type of calibrator (pistonphone), designed by Dunn and Rahm, provided an independent and absolute source of calibration. Both systems were used for calibration of microphones, not for direct calibration of the vibrations recorded from patients. The same applies to the calibrators of Mannheimer and of Yoshimura.

CALIBRATION OF AMPLIFIER AND FILTER

One type of calibrator was used by the Sanborn Company in the Stetho-Cardiette and in the Twin-Beam. Its principle is the following: The compression of a button gives an electric sine wave of 60 hz, which is recorded with a magnitude comparable to that of a sound of 90 db taking place within the microphone. Unfortunately, this low-pitched signal was attenuated by the filter used in logarithmic phonocardiography. Later Wells *et al.* (1949) employed a signal of 500 hz and 80 db for calibrating aortic diastolic murmurs. Similar calibrators, based on a 50 hz signal, were used by Yoshimura, by Ueda and Sakamoto* (either 1 or 5 mV), and by Sloan and Greer (2.4 mV).

It is obvious that these calibrators give only a gross idea of the degree of amplification, which is then altered by the response

---

*Zalter *et al.* (1963) calibrated various microphones in the following way: An artificial surface closely resembling the chest wall was constructed. A close approximation was found empirically by mounting a 6-mm layer of soft sponge rubber on a rigid platform and covering this with chamois skin treated with a light coat of sealant. The artificial skin and the microphone were placed on a vibrating platform driven by an electric oscillator. The vibratory amplitude was monitored by an accelerometer connected to an electric voltmeter. The displacement amplitude was measured by a microscope using a strobscope light to illuminate the surface. The output voltage of the microphone was determined while a known voltage was supplied in series with it. A combination of these two data gave the open-circuit voltage response of the microphone.

*Personal communication.

of the filter system. In addition, the following factors should be considered:

1. Changes resulting from a different thickness of the air cushion (lung tissue) interposed between the heart and chest wall are important. The latter may easily vary because of a different phase of apnea and may further vary because of pathologic changes of the lungs (emphysema or sclerosis) or the pleura (fibrosis, effusion).

2. Changes resulting from different thickness of the chest wall and its surrounding tissues are particularly important if the microphone is even slightly displaced from its initial position, and particularly so in females (left breast).

3. Changes resulting from different pressures of the air contained in the bell of a microphone are caused by different degrees of tension of the rubber strap or, to a lesser extent, by the addition of a side chamber (recording of both a phonocardiogram and an apex cardiogram).

Bernstein and I have developed an electric calibrator. A signal of 800 hz was applied to the Sanborn amplifier with two alternative magnitudes corresponding to either 1 mV or 10 mV. These magnitudes covered the entire frequency range and gave a signal that was within the width of the recording film when the desired amplification of sounds was obtained. The 800 hz signal passed unattenuated by the various high-pass filters and, therefore, was suitable for any of the used bands. In spite of its obvious limitations, this calibrator proved useful, especially in comparing sounds from two different microphones.

CALIBRATION OF MICROPHONE, AMPLIFIER, AND FILTER

Bernstein and I have developed a new sound calibrator that consists of a tiny sound generator (like those used in hearing aids) applied to the bell of a dynamic microphone and connected to an oscillator. An 800 hz sound signal of between 1 and 10 volts acts on the microphone and is recorded as a sine wave on the tracing. This signal is modified by the tension of the rubber strap holding the dynamic microphone in place, by the characteristics of the microphone and amplifier, and by the degree of amplification. The smaller voltage is used for high-frequency tracings requiring great amplification, and vice versa. The highest intensity of the signal is about 45 db.

This calibrator cannot be employed for apparatus using band pass filters because the high-frequency signal would be modified by the low-pass section of the filter. In such equipment, the frequency of the signal should be modified so that it would match that of the nominal frequency of the filter. This can be done by moving a special rheostat of the oscillator.

Another sound calibrator was developed in our laboratory, prompted by the observation that various sound generators for hearing aids give sounds of different magnitudes. This model consists of a loudspeaker mounted on the ceiling of the sound proof chamber 1 meter from the patient's chest. It is connected to a small amplifier and to an oscillator. The latter sends an 800 hz signal of between 0.1 and 10 volts to the loudspeaker. The system permits us to calibrate either one or two microphones on the chest, and can be used for any type of microphone including

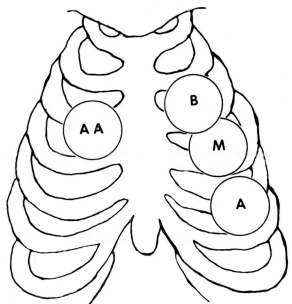

FIGURE 50. The main phonocardiographic areas and one of the auxiliary areas of the precordium. A = apex; M = midprecordium; B = base; AA = ascending aortic area.

the contact type. The sound signal was measured as being between 45 and 95 db at the microphone.

OUR PRESENT CALIBRATORS

In our present set up, we have two systems used for calibration. The first is a self-contained unit for making accurate field calibrations of microphones. It generates a single note sound at a known sound pressure level with five preferred frequencies. Each of them can be used so that sensitivity and response tests can be made at several frequencies. The second is an electric signal output built in the preamplifier. This will be used for calibrating amplification, filter action, and differentiation circuits for frequencies from 10 to 1000 hz. The microphone itself is independent of pressure changes in its application to the chest.

CLINICAL-INSTRUMENTAL CALIBRATION

Luisada and Gamna attempted to effect clinical calibration by applying a sound signal of known frequency and amplitude to the chest wall (the best location was the margin of the left pectoral muscle). This crude system proved to be of a certain value in evaluating the damping effect of lung tissue or pleural fluid, as well as the effect of varying the tension of the rubber strap.

Heintzen and Vietor have attempted to calibrate cardiac sound by applying a standard sound signal of various frequencies to the precordium and recording it intracardially by means of a phonocatheter. Even though this method is of interest for scientific investigations, it does not lend itself to practical application because of the need for an intracardiac sound recorder. The same can be said for the sound calibrator of Feruglio. He introduced sound into the heart by means of a sound generator attached to a catheter closed at the tip by a membrane. The vibrations were picked up by the standard microphone applied to the precordium. This system extended the method used by Zalter *et al.* (1963) in animals and may prove to be of interest for animal research and clinical investigation in spite of some artifacts inherent in the system.*

A modification of this system has been attempted by Feruglio; it consists of the introduction of sound into the esopha-

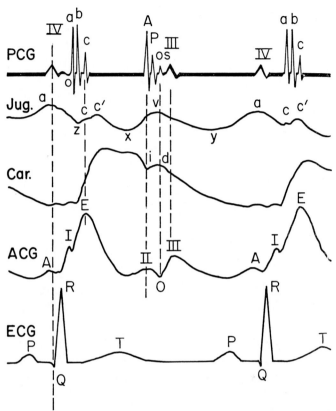

FIGURE 51. Scheme of the correlations of the phonocardiographic deflections with those of the auxiliary clinical tracings.

gus during the recording of a phonocardiogram. If accurate, this method would record a sound vibration modified by all variables (physiologic, anatomic, and instrumental) except for those related to the structure and functional state of the cardiac walls. It might prove of considerable scientific interest, even though it would not be suitable for routine use.

*The amplitude of the vibrations is affected by the pressure exerted by the heart on the membrane of the catheter (personal tests). Therefore, accurate comparison can be made only during diastole. It is interesting to note that Heintzen's method also reveals a different modulation of the sound amplitude according to the chamber in which the signal is recorded. If technical artifacts are excluded, this might reveal a *different transmission by the contracting (in comparison with the relaxed) cardiac wall.* This fact might be one of the factors of the generally greater amplitude of systolic, in comparison with diastolic, murmurs.

Chapter 18

Intracardiac Phonocardiography

FOLLOWING the pioneering works of Yamakawa *et al.*, and Soulié, Luisada and Liu (1957) described a method of recording intracardiac sound vibrations utilizing the electric signal of a high frequency pressure transducer through differentiation and filtration. At the same time, Lewis *et al.* (1957) used a miniature barium titanate tubular element at the tip of an intracardiac catheter for recording sound vibrations. More recently Soulié *et al.* (1959, 1961) published the results of their studies with a pressure-sound transducer placed at the tip of a catheter (micromanometer).

Numerous studies of intracardiac phonocardiography have been published (Feruglio, Yamakawa, Moscovitz *et al.*, 1958, 1963). Some of them dealt primarily with animal studies or investigation of the right heart, and a few reported occasional studies of the left heart. Others (Liu *et al.*, Luisada and Liu, 1958) dealt specifically with investigations of the left atrium and ventricle, and of the aorta. A study by Yarza Iriarte *et al.*, used a modification* of Luisada and Liu's method in 38 patients with congenital heart disease and in 20 patients with acquired heart disease. Soulié *et al.* (1961) reported the data obtained in a few cases in which patients were studied by left heart catheterization.

---

*A piezoelectric microphone was cemented to the end of the catheter. A similar method was also used by Faber and Purvis for experimental investigations.

Kasparian *et al.* studied several patients by catheterization of the left ventricle.

Since 1956, we have used two different methods to obtain an automatic recording of the sound phenomena during the diagnostic procedure of catheterization. These permitted us to draw blood samples from the catheter and to avoid the introduction of additional catheters. Moreover, difficulty in the positioning of phonocatheters (especially in the left heart) and frequent damage of the sensor element is avoided by this method. These advantages were partially offset in the first method by the fact that high-frequency vibrations were poorly recorded, partly because they were above the response limit of the strain gauge, and partly because of damping caused by the catheter* (Fig. 52).

The first method, already described, was based on the electric output of a strain gauge. The second method, more recently developed, was based on the application of a flat, sonar-type, barium titanate microphone at the end of a catheter. In this, the vibrations of the blood within the chambers of the heart and vessels were transmitted along the fluid of the catheter and transduced by the microphone (Luisada *et al.*, 1965). This system, called an FCT** phonocardiogram, proved adequate for low-frequency vibrations and is excellent for high-frequency vibrations.***

Sound vibrations travel in water with a speed of 1,500 m per sec.; thus, the rapid intracardiac vibrations reach the strain gauge pickup with a delay of 0.7 meec. A further delay is introduced by the electronic differentiation and filtration, so that an actual delay of 5 to 10 msec. can be observed in the tracings recorded from a strain guage in comparison with external phonocardiograms. Our modification of the original method suggested by Yarza Iriarte *et al.* has the advantage that it increases the

---

*An objection voiced in the past stated that the high-frequency vibrations derived from the signal of the pressure transducer were different phenomena from the heart sounds and murmurs. This objection has gradually lost its validity because studies of the last decade (Faber and Purvis, Piemme and Dexter, and Dexter) have revealed that the main vibrations of the heart sounds coincide in time with the rapid rises and drops of the pressure tracings, confirming that they can be derived from the latter through differentiation.

**"Fluid column transmission" system.

***A similar system has been used by Guenther and the results are described in his book (1969).

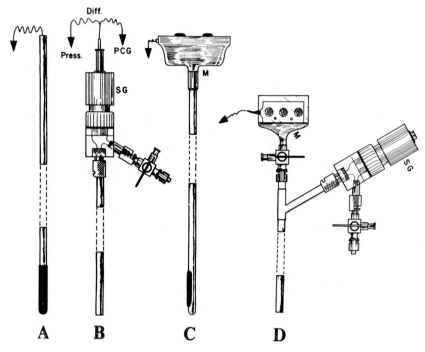

FIGURE 52. Intracardiac microphones. (A) Phonocatheters (Allard-Laurens, SF1). (B) Strain gauge with electric differentiation (Luisada-Liu). (C) Catheter closed by membrane (Feruglio). (D) Strain gauge (Sg) and fluid transmission microphone (m) (Luisada-Slodki).

frequency response of the system and decreases the delay, so that the medium high-frequency vibrations are recorded with fidelity.

Analysis of the intracardiac phonocardiogram was made by Luisada *et al.* (1964) in 172 clinical cases in which patients were subjected to catheterization of the right heart, left heart, or both, including 34 patients with minimal or no hemodynamic alterations (Fig. 53).

Even though the vibrations equivalent to heart sounds and murmurs are largest in the chamber, and near the valve or shunt, in which they originate, they can also be recorded in other chambers or vessels. The right ventricle and the pulmonary artery receive and transmit vibrations originating in the left heart or aorta. Wedge tracings of the left lung record left heart vibrations.

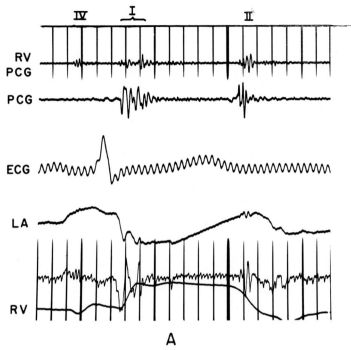

FIGURE 53. Intracardiac phonocardiogram from right ventricle (A), left atrium (B), pulmonary artery (C), and aorta (D). Case with insignificant mitral stenosis.

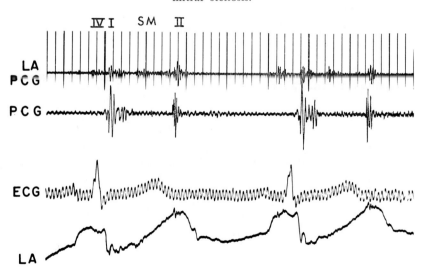

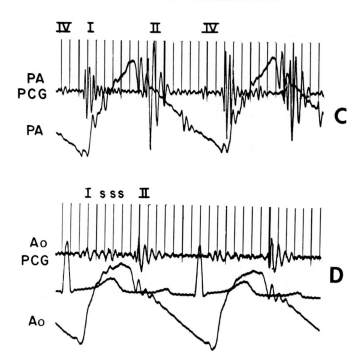

The latter are also recorded in the right atrium whenever they are large or the ascending aorta is dilated.

A study was also made of the atrial and third sounds, of the early and late (ejection) components of the first sound, of the aortic and pulmonary components of the second sound, of the opening sound or snap of the AV valves, and of various murmurs.

The great intensity of the murmur of mitral insufficiency on the atrial side of the mitral valve (with limited transmission to the ventricle) and the presence of the murmur of mitral stenosis in the left ventricle (with little transmission to the atrium) were confirmed.

The greatest intensity of the murmur of ventricular septal defect on the right side of the shunt, that of the murmur of patent ductus arteriosus in the ductus itself and (to a lesser extent) in the pulmonary artery, and that of the systolic murmur of atrial septal defect in the pulmonary artery (pulmonary flow murmur) were also confirmed.

The small aortic component of the second sound in aortic

stenosis and the small pulmonary component of the second sound in pulmonary stenosis are usually well recorded in the respective artery, thus aiding in their identification. The murmur of diffuse narrowing of the pulmonary vessels is well recorded peripherally, much more than that of pulmonary stenosis.

In conclusion, intracardiac phonocardiography should be considered as a method of great diagnostic value in cases of rheumatic heart disease and of congenital heart disease. It is of aid in obscure cases of myocardopathy or coronary heart disease with extra-sounds or murmurs.

Chapter 19

Other Special Phonocardiographic Techniques

FETAL PHONOCARDIOGRAM

TRACINGS of fetal sounds were recorded by Pestalozza in 1891. Since then, many researchers have published fetal tracings with a gradually improving technique (Sampson *et al.,* Beruti; Hyman: Peralta; Ramos; Lian and Golblin; Pereira; Cesa and Seganti; Jordan and Randolph; Luisada, 1953; and Fishleder, 1960).

Fetal phonocardiography is easier than fetal electrocardiography. It permits evaluation of the rate of the fetal heart and may even make possible prenatal diagnosis of congenital heart disease (Jordan and Randolph).

The microphone with a large chest piece is applied over that part of the maternal abdomen where auscultation reveals fetal heart sounds. Simultaneous with the fetal phonocardiogram, a maternal electrocardiogram is recorded. Comparison of the tracings proves whether or not the sounds auscultated were fetal heart sounds.

Bolechowski *et al.* recorded routinely fetal heart sounds after the twentieth week of pregnancy in 164 women. The best records were obtained in the frequency bands above 35 hz. In addition to fetal heart sounds, umbilical cord murmur, noise caused by movement of the fetus, and the maternal souffle were recorded.

In tracings that I have recorded, the fetal sounds were registered in all bands from 15 to 500 hz. The best tracings, however, were in the lower (50 or 100 hz) bands (Fig. 54). In passing from the low to the high bands, the first heart sound becomes attenuated, like in the adult tracing. Thus, at 200 or 400 hz, only one sound (usually the second) is visible.

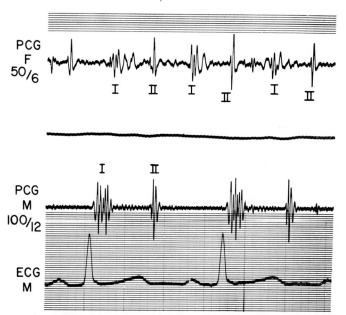

FIGURE 54. Fetal electrocardiogram. *From above:* —Fetal electrocardiogram at 6 months of pregnancy. —Maternal phonocardiogram. —Maternal electrocardiogram.

Smaller vibrations are also recorded. The most common are (1) a small, low-pitched, early systolic vibration; (2) a small third sound; and (3) more rarely, a small fourth sound.

ESOPHAGEAL PHONOCARDIOGRAPHY

Extensive studies with esophageal phonocardiography have been made by Taquini (1937) and, later, by Miller and Groedel. The interest of the method lies in the fact that the heart sounds are collected from inside the chest: Their origin is near the collecting chamber, and their transmission is not altered by bony structures.

The first component of the fourth sound is often recorded, so that the fourth sound takes place earlier than at the apex, where only a subsequent component is recorded.

The phonocardiogram is recorded by using a stomach tube closed at the end by a rubber membrane or small balloon. The most interesting tracing is that obtained at the atrial level, i.e., at 45 cm from the teeth or nostrils in an adult (Fig. 55). Atrial sounds and the murmur caused by mitral insufficiency are more distinctly recorded than from the surface of the chest. Sounds

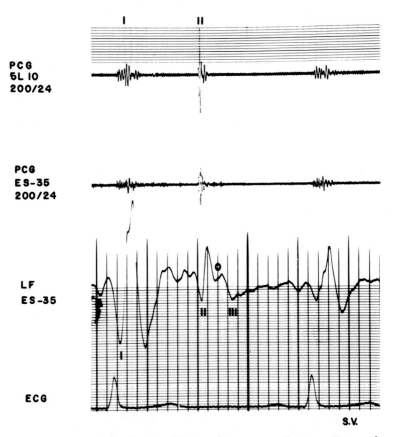

FIGURE 55. Esophageal phonocardiogram in a normal man. *From above:* High frequency tracing recorded over the apex; esophageal high frequency tracing at 35 cm; esophageal low frequency tracing at 35 cm; electrocardiogram.

and murmurs may have lower frequencies than when recorded by the conventional technique.

A more modern method is based on recording the phonocardiogram by means of a specially constructed piezoelectric, catheter-tip transducer.

TRACHEAL PHONOCARDIOGRAPHY

Tracheal phonocardiograms have been recorded in patients having a tracheal cannula by Groedel and Miller. The technique consists of connecting the outer end of the cannula with a microphone by means of a short piece of rubber tube. The heart sounds are shorter and have vibrations of lower frequency than when they are recorded from outside the chest.

EPICARDIC PHONOCARDIOGRAM

The phonocardiogram can be recorded directly from the epicardium of the exposed heart or the adventitia of the large vessels. Several authors recorded such tracings in animals (Bertrand *et al.,* Zalter *et al.,* 1963, Shah *et al.,* 1963A) and in man (Magri *et al.*). The tracings are recorded by means of a double-rim funnel, which is kept adherent to the cardiac surface by a continuous suction device.

The intensity of the heart sounds is several times greater on the heart than on the precordium, and the low frequency vibrations are particularly well recorded by this method.

A modification of the method has been recently suggested by Groom (personal communication). By means of a special device and an airtight well, the sounds can be recorded without actual contact with the heart. This method is of interest because it avoids artifacts due to the cardiac motion even though it may introduce others as a result of the shifting of the heart mass.

Chapter 20

Standardization and Nomenclature

Standardization

PHONOCARDIOGRAPHY still suffers from lack of uniformity both in regard to apparatus and to interpretation of the tracings.

An *International Committee on Standardization* held two meetings, one in 1950 (First World Congress of Cardiology) and the other in 1953 .(Meeting of La Société Francaise de Cardiologie). Their conclusions were published in 1955* One suggestion gave instructions regarding the notation of the area of recording. This should be noted with an Arabic numeral for the intercostal space, followed by a capital letter indicating whether it is right or left (R or L), followed by another Arabic numeral indicating the number of centimeters from the midsternal line. (Example: 3L6 means the third left inter space at 6 cm from the midsternal line.)

At that time agreement was reached on the fact that the basic phonocardiographic tracing should follow the sensitivity curve of the human ear. The possibility of recording two other tracings was considered, however, one for vibrations of lower frequency and the other for vibrations of higher frequency. This

---

*See Kleyn *et al.,* 1955.

obviously would require the use of (additional) * filters.

A third meeting was held in connection with the Second European Congress of Cardiology (Stockholm, 1956) and the conclusions were published in 1957.** The scope of phono-cardiography was considerably enlarged, and the use of several channels was advocated. Definition of the nominal frequency was given. Intervals of one octave between channels were considered advisable.

During the Third World Congress of Cardiology (Brussels, 1958), several participants held a meeting dealing with technical problems of phonocardiography.

The representatives of the various countries agreed that it would be premature to establish definite frequency characteristics to be used in the construction of phonocardiographs.

The following points were accepted:†

1. It is necessary to use some type of filter in order to obtain relevant and clinically significant phonocardiographic tracings.

2. If the frequency response given by microphone, amplifiers, and recording units is linear (a highly desirable feature of an apparatus), the most important variable is represented by the filter or filters. The frequency response of all these parts, including filters, should be such as to give the desired response for each frequency.

3. It would be desirable for each researcher to indicate in his publications the frequency characteristics of his filters in a uniform manner.

   (a) When only a high-pass filter is used, the researcher should give a series of Arabic numerals separated by fraction lines. The first number denotes the frequency at which the increase in amplitude reaches 10 per cent (or —20 db) of the maximum value. The second number indicates the slope reached at

---

*This word was added because obviously no apparatus would record a curve similar to that of the ear without some method of electric or mechanical filtration.

**See Mannheimer, 1957.

†See Kleyn *et al.,* 1959.

this point in db per octave. (Example: 140
(—20db) /24.)

(b) When a band-pass filter is used, the researcher should
indicate in the same way the frequency characteristics
for both the high-pass and the low-pass filters; the
figures of the two filters should be separated by a
horizontal line. (Example: 140 (—20db) /24 —500
(—20db) /24.)

After this meeting, an exchange of letters took place prompted by the observation that the foregoing description failed to
indicate the most desirable characteristics of high-pass or band-
pass filters with a peaked circuit. It was then agreed that two
points would be sufficient for such description, the —3 db and
the —20 db point.

Each researcher was left free to select the most suitable
bands.

A new meeting was held at the Fourth World Congress of
Cardiology (Mexico City, 1962). Several committees were ap-
pointed, including one on standardization and one on nomencla-
ture. Further discussion on nomenclature took place at the III
Asian-Pacific Congress of Cardiology (Kyoto, 1964). The con-
clusions of the various committees were presented at the Third
European Congress of Cardiology (Prague, 1964 published by
Holldack *et al.,* 1965).

NOMENCLATURE

Phonocardiogram

The report presented in Prague (1964) suggested the following rules.

Designation of the tracing. The phonocardiographic tracing
will be designated by the symbol PCG.

Area of recording. The intercostal space will be indicated
by an Arabic numeral. The capital letters R or L will indicate
the right or left side, and the distance in centimeters from the
midsternal line will be designated by an Arabic numeral.*
(Examples: 4L7; 5R4.) In addition, 4S would designate the
sternum at the level of the fourth space. The designation "apex"

---

*This designation had been approved by a previous International Committee for
Standardization.

indicates that a particular area coincides with the point of maximal impulse.

These symbols will be marked in the margin at the left of the tracing.

Phase of respiration. The symbols *Insp.* and *Exp.* designate inspiratory and expiratory apnea, respectively. The symbol *Resp.* designates the tracing if the patient is breathing normally.

These designations should be placed in the margin below those indicating the area of recording.

Characteristics of equipment. If the apparatus makes use of a high-pass filter, one should use the notation corresponding to the nominal frequency in hz over a fraction line, and that corresponding to the slope in db under such line. (Examples: 30/6, 100/12, 400/24.) ** This will be designated in the margin.

Phases of cardiac cycle. Systole will be indicated by the capital letter S, and diastole by the capital letter D.

Heart sounds. The heart sounds should should be indicated by the roman numerals I, II, III, and IV, which should be marked above the sounds.

First sound. The letters *a, b, c,* and *d* should be used to designate the major groups of vibrations. To designate the ejection sound separately, the capital letter E should be used.

(Example: $\dfrac{\mathrm{I}}{a, b, c, d, E}$.)

Second sound. The capital letters A and P will designate the

aortic and pulmonary components.* (Example: $\dfrac{\mathrm{II}}{AP}$.)

Third sound. The third heart sound should be designated by the roman numeral III without reference to the ventricle of origin. The latter may be surmised from the area of recording. If there are different components, they should be called a, b, and

---

** More complex and accurate ways of noting have been mentioned in the previous section.

---

*The reason for using capital letters instead of lower case letters (like those for the first sound) is that they should designate the origin of the component and not the sequence of events. Thus, a paradoxical or reverse splitting will be designated as P.A.

c. (Example: $\dfrac{\text{III}}{\text{a, b, c}}$.)

Fourth sound. The fourth heart sound should be designated by the Roman numeral IV including cases of AV block. If there are several components of the sound, lower case letters can be

used. (Example: $\dfrac{\text{IV}}{\text{a, b, c}}$.)

In cases of triple rhythms and quadruple rhythms, the same designations III and IV will be placed over the respective sounds if recognizable. (Example I, II, III, or I, II, III, IV) If there is fusion or summation of III and IV, the symbol will be $\dfrac{\text{III}}{\text{IV}}$ or III-IV.

Opening snap. The opening snap will be designated simply as OS. Any indication of whether it is mitral or tricuspid, physiologic or pathologic, should be given in the legend or text or may be surmised from the area of best recording.

Clicks. Both the pathologic clicks and those originating in a prosthetic valve will be designated as K. However, for the latter, mitral closure click is indicated as MC, mitral opening, as MO; aortic closure click is indicated as AC, and aortic opening, as AO. The pericardial knock will be designated as K.

Pericardial friction rubs. Each main group will be designated as F or FR. The fact that a particular group of vibrations is in systole or diastole is obvious on inspection of the tracing but can be designated as SR or DR.

Murmurs. A murmur will be designated as M. The following symbols should be used: presystolic murmur — PM; diastolic murmur — DM; systolic murmur — SM.

Any further description of phase and configuration should be given in the legend or text.

Any *extraneous noise* (borborygmus, rhonchus, rale) will be designated as X.

Ultralow-frequency tracing

Nomenclature of the waves of an ultralow-frequency tracing (apex cardiogram, epigastric cardiogram, kinetocardiogram) still escapes international agreement, partly due to different instrumentation.

One system of description (Luisada, 1953) has been partly followed by others. It will be summarized here.

Considering the unitary nature of the precordial vibration phenomenon, the waves of a mechanical tracing should be correlated as much as possible with those of any other. As certain groups of vibrations (sounds I, II, III, and IV) are sharper and better visible in medium-frequency tracings, they can be taken as landmarks, and similar symbols can be given to the waves of the ULF tracing. The first rapid rise will be I; the second systolic peak will be E (ejection). The notch ending the systolic collapse will be II; the wave of rapid filling will be III,* the presystolic wave will be IV. There is another notch that is fairly constant and significant. It is usually of negative polarity, is intermediate between II and III, and most likely coincides with the opening of the mitral valve. For this reason it has been suggested to call this notch point σ (opening of valve).

It should be kept in mind that occasionally an inverted polarity of all or most waves may occur.

---

*British authors have called this wave "F," from "filling."

Part VI

ROUTINE PHONOCARDIOGRAPHIC STUDY

Chapter 21

Phonocardiographic Areas

ROUTINE PROCEDURE

THE PROBLEM of how to study the vibrations of the pre-cordium has fundamental theoretical implications because it is based on the underlying philosophy of the final aims of phonocardiography. Phonocardiography is so intimately connected with physical examination, on the one hand, and with technical problems, on the other, that it may be practised according to different viewpoints and with different results.

There is no question that—in phonocardiography as in other methods of study of a cardiac patient—the greater the skill, the maturity, and the patience of the observer, the more satisfactory and complete will be the results.

Certain physicians are dissatisfied with the phonocardiograph because they cannot leave it, as they can with an electrocardiograph, in the hands of a technician. This is not altogether true. A technician can be trained in about a year so that he can record satisfactory tracings. However, the data gathered by him will not be as important or illuminating as those obtained by a trained cardiologist.

In our experience with training persons at various levels, the necessary time for technical training is grossly as follows:

1. An able and interested technician can be trained in about a year.

2. A physician at the Resident level can be trained in 6 months.
3. An internist with an interest in cardiology and some theoretical background can be trained in a month.

This listing alone indicates that the answers obtained in the last two cases will be more extensive and complete than in the first case, where a standardized and automatic system of study is likely to be developed without reference to the specific problems of the individual patient.

The moderate clinical experience of the Resident and the practically absent clinical experience of the technician can be partly compensated for if the patient is sent prepared for the study with: (1) a tentative diagnosis; (2) a description of sounds or murmurs to be studied; and (3) markings on the skin of the locations where such phenomena are heard best.

Obviously, this requires a close collaboration between the hospital and laboratory staffs. If such is lacking (the overworked Residents of a modern hospital seldom have time for such collaboration), the only alternative is to have the physician in charge of the phonocardiogram take a complete history and perform a physical examination, which should be exhaustive in regard to the cardiovascular system. On the basis of his findings, he will then proceed to the technical study of the patient. The recorded phonocardiograms are then discussed at a Phonocardiography Conference, where all clinical, electrocardiographic, and roentgenologic data are presented and where senior cardiologists contribute, not only to the descriptive interpretation of the tracings, but also to their clinical evaluation.

GENERAL INSTRUCTIONS

Phonocardiograms can be recorded in any room, provided that a reasonably low noise level can be obtained. I have recorded fair tracings in private homes and hospital wards. In both cases one should ask patients, relatives, and nurses to maintain complete silence during the recording.

In a hospital, a quiet laboratory is often difficult to find. Obviously, *a special room should be devoted to phonocardiography*. If possible, the room should be *soundproofed* and provided with a thick door. If conventional soundproofing with tiles is not possible, draperies along the wall and over the door can obtain the same results.

Another possibility is that of building a *small, air conditioned, soundproof chamber* within the laboratory of phonocardiography (Fig. 49). Since this does not require complete soundproofing, construction can be made at moderate cost.

Whenever the phonocardiograph has a noisy fan, its motion should be discontinued during the taking of a record by pressing a foot switch.

The following scheme of examination is based on the working procedure used in our laboratory. Obviously, it should be modified if different equipment is used, special research is contemplated, or special clinical problems are investigated.

In reading this scheme of study, one should keep in mind that the following description is intended only as a guide. The location of the microphone should be modified if needed (greater amplitude or different characteristics of a sound or murmur in an atypical location).

PHONOCARDIOGRAPHIC AREAS

In our laboratory, chest pieces of 3.5 cm diameter are used both in large animals and man.

Experience has shown us that three main areas should be used in the routine study of a patient (Fig. 50).

1. *The apical area.* This area centers on the point of maximum impulse. If such impulse is not visible or felt, the microphone is applied at the midclavicular line over the 4th and 5th intercostal spaces. It will reveal most mitral murmurs (especially those related to mitral insufficiency), the first, third, and fourth sounds, occasionally the tricuspid murmurs (if the right heart is extremely dilated), and sometimes the aortic murmurs.

2. *The midprecordial area.* This area is at the center of the precordium, between sternum and apex, over the 3rd and 4th intercostal spaces. It reveals best the configuration of the first and second sounds, the opening snap, the murmur of mitral stenosis, that of tricuspid stenosis or

insufficiency, the murmur of ventricular septal defect, the murmurs of aortic stenosis (especially the muscular type) and aortic insufficiency, the murmur of pulmonic insufficiency. Less well is recorded the murmur of pulmonic stenosis.

3. *The area of the base.* This area centers on the 2nd left interspace about 5-6 cm from the midsternal line. It reveals best the configuration and splitting of the second sound, the murmurs of pulmonic stenosis and insufficiency, those of aortic stenosis and insufficiency and of patent ductus arteriosus, occasionally that of mitral insufficiency and that of ventricular septal defect.

Certain auxiliary areas should be used in particular cases:

(a) If the heart is severely enlarged to the left, a tracing should be recorded *over the 6th left i.c.s.* This will particularly reveal *mitral murmurs.*

(b) If the heart is severely enlarged to the right, a tracing should be recorded *over the 4th-5th right i.c.s* close to the sternum. This will particularly reveal tricuspid murmurs and the murmur of ventricular septal defect.

(c) *The ascending aortic area.* If the ascending aorta is dilated, one should record a tracing over the 2nd and 3rd right i.c.s. close to the sternum. This will reveal aortic murmurs, especially that of aortic stenosis (Fig. 50).

(d) *The first left i.c.s.* This is best for recording the murmur of patent ductus arteriosus.

(e) *Lateral chest areas.* These are used for murmurs of pulmonic branches coarctation.

(f) *Posterior areas.* These are used for recording the murmur of aortic coarctation.

Whenever a murmur is heard over an unusual location, a tracing should be recorded over that area.

In certain cases, the manubrium of the sternum or the suprasternal notch may reveal faint aortic murmurs, especially if the aortic arch is dilated.

Tracings can be recorded over the cervical areas, the flanks, the anterior aspect of the neck, the femoral areas or the epigastrium for recording peripheral vascular murmurs.

ROUTINE PROCEDURE

Step 1

As soon as the patient arrives in the department, he is taken to the *ECG room* for a routine tracing.

Step 2

He is then transferred to the *Phono room* and seated in a chair, where routine history is taken and physical examination is performed including blood pressure measurement.

Step 3

The patient is placed on the bed of the *sound-proof chamber* and asked to relax.* The electrodes are applied to the limbs, and a rapid check is made with the stethoscope for the best location of murmurs and extra sounds. Then the microphone is applied in succession over the various areas.

For each of the locations, one should check the oscilloscope tracing and adjust the amplification until either the heart sounds or the murmurs (if these are very large) have an amplitude of 3-5 cm (velocity tracing). At this time, a tape recording is made of the PCG and ECG while no filter is used.

One should write in the book of *Protocols* the figure of the tape spool indicating the beginning of the record, and one should make a voice announcement of the patient's name, the location of microphone, and the type of recording. For each tracing recorded on tape, the protocol should also indicate the degree of attenuation of *preamplifier* and *amplifier*.

In patients with low frequency sounds (gallops), a *displacement tracing* will also be recorded through the band pass filter at 0-100. In patients with high frequency murmurs, an *acceleration tracing* can also be recorded.

Step 4

Following completion of these records, optional tracings may be taken at the apex or base in the left decubitus or in the sitting position. All these tracings are taken with normal respiration after instructing the patient to breathe slowly and shallowly.

---

*In infants and young children, complete relaxation is often impossible without sedation. In such cases, a Nembutal suppository (0.1 gm) is introduced into the rectum. The tracings are recorded when the effect becomes apparent, from 45 to 60 minutes later.

Should the patient have noisy respiration, then the tracing should be recorded in expiratory apnea. A tracing of respiration is simultaneously recorded by using a special bellows connected to a linear microphone.

Following these recordings, *precordial motions* are recorded in apnea with the pickup placed first at the apex, and then at any other point of the precordium where a visible or palpable motion is observed. Then a *carotid pulse tracing* and a *jugular pulse tracing* are tape-recorded in succession together with ECG and PCG. In cases with an enlarged liver, a *hepatogram* is also recorded, again with ECG and PCG.

Step 5

We now proceed to the *drug tests* (see later). Patients with a pansystolic murmur at apex or midprecordium should receive *Methoxamine*. Patients with a loud and harsh systolic murmur at the base should receive first *amyl nitrite,* and 15 minutes later *Isuprel*. The others should receive only *amyl nitrite*. The microphone should be placed over the area of the most significant murmur before performing the test.

Drug test tracings will be recorded on tape with a filtration of 0-400.

At this point the patient can be dismissed. Then transcription is made from the tape to the phonocardiographic film.* The velocity phonocardiogram, which had been recorded without any filter, is now passed through the band pass filter, and three filtered recordings are made for each location as well as for the drug test:

0-100;   50-400;   200-800**

Amplification is made before recording, and is checked on the oscilloscope, so that the final tracing will show heart sounds or murmurs of about 3-5 cm of amplitude.

Note should be taken that, in passing from a lower to a higher filtration, the amplification will need to be increased.

In our laboratory, the phonocardiograms are often recorded in expiratory apnea, this being defined as the position reached

---

*The tape is rewound to the initial figure and then transcription is made.

**If 200-800 does not yield a good tracing, 100-800 will be taken instead. In the case of a very high pitched murmur, a higher frequency band can be recorded.

after normal expiration. A brief instruction to the patient precedes the first tracing. The subject is advised to breathe normally and to hold his breath in the desired position upon request of the operator or flashing of a light signal.

Chapter 22

Functional Tests

CARDIOACTIVE AND VASOACTIVE DRUGS

Respiration

THE MOST PHYSIOLOGICAL test in phonocardiography is represented by normal or forced respiration. Inspiration increases venous return to the right heart and increases pulmonary blood flow; it decreases for a brief time the flow to the left heart, Expiration has the opposite effect. Inspiration widens the splitting of the second sound in most subjects. Exceptions are represented by cases with atrial septal defect or right bundle branch block in whom the modifications are minimal (wide, fixed splitting).

Murmurs originating in the right heart chambers or pulmonary artery are said to increase during inspiration while those originating in the left heart chambers or aorta are said to increase during expiration. This fact was noted long ago in regard to murmurs caused by tricuspid lesions; the same concept was later extended to murmurs caused by pulmonary valve lesions and to flow murmurs of the pulmonary artery. It is unfortunate that, as the vibrations caused by respiratory sound are within the frequency range of cardiac sound, the phonocardiogram obtained during respiration is often unrevealing in regard to heart sounds and murmurs. This is particularly true for records obtained with the microphone placed over the areas of the base while tracings recorded at the apex or midprecordium often have sufficient clarity for being significant. On the other hand, the ear is often able to discriminate between heart murmurs and the respiratory murmurs. Therefore, respiratory tests are often more revealing if performed as an office or bedside procedure.

The most significant data that can be observed during respiration are (a) variations in the degree of splitting of the second sound, and (b) changes in the magnitude of murmurs.

The respiration record can be obtained: (1) by means of a bellow wrapped around the waistline and connected with a crystal microphone with linear response; it is recorded with a DC amplifier; (2) by introducing a bakelite olive in one of the nostrils; this is again connected to the same microphone and amplifier.

Both tracings inscribe small waves caused by the heart and vessels and large, slower deflections due to respiration. The polarity of the recorder should be such that inspiration is revealed by a drop of the tracing.

If no reliable data are obtained by this method, one can record two phonocardiograms in succession, one in *inspiratory apnea* and the other in *expiratory apnea*. The changes of sounds and murmurs occurring at the beginning of each phase are similar to those caused by normal respiration but are often less marked.

Among the important use of respiration as a functional test, it should be mentioned that *right-sided murmurs* in general and *tricuspid murmurs* in particular are increased by inspiration. The murmur of atrial septal defect and that of pulmonary stenosis are also larger in inspiration. *Left-sided murmurs* in general, and mitral murmurs in particular, are larger in expiration. The murmur of ventricular septal defect is also larger in expiration. See also Footnote at the end of Chap. 24.

Valsalva Maneuver

Zinsser and Kay suggested the use of the Valsalva maneuver for the study of cardiovascular alterations. Numerous authors have investigated the dynamic changes resulting from this maneuver (Sarnoff *et al.*, 1948, Sharpey-Schafer, Wood, 1956, Zinsser and Kay, Polis *et al.*, Fishleder, 1963).

The following changes have been observed. During the straining procedure, all murmurs are decreased because of decreased venous return and lower cardiac output. As soon as straining is terminated (15 to 30 sec.), the murmurs originating in the right heart increase whereas those originating in the left heart increase much later (30 to 90 sec.).

Unfortunately, this maneuver requires active participation of the patient. It cannot be used in children less than 6 to 8 years of age; it should *not* be used in patients with coronary or cerebral arteriosclerosis; it is difficult to perform if the patient has dyspnea; and it is incorrectly performed by uncooperative or poorly alert patients. Moreover, the severity of the straining will vary from case to case. For these reasons, this test is not currently employed in our laboratory.

Cardioactive and Vasoactive Drugs

The possibility of surgical correction of congenital abnormalities and acquired valvular lesions has increased the interest of auscultation as one of the most important diagnostic methods. Even though cardiac catheterization and angiocardiography are often used in the final evaluation of certain cases, not all patients are submitted to these procedures. Therefore, auscultation and its technical counterpart (phonocardiography) have basic importance among the physical and technical diagnostic methods.

Phonocardiography supplies information concerning magnitude of heart sounds, splitting of heart sounds, presence of additional systolic or diastolic sounds, and the characteristics of murmurs. All these data are usually collected while the patient is at rest and cardiac output is at a relatively low level. It is obvious that the heart sounds and the murmurs are modified by changes in heart rate, blood pressure, and blood flow. This is why several drugs have been employed in the study of murmurs in order to improve the accuracy of diagnosis and for differential diagnosis.

EFFECT OF DRUGS ON HEMODYNAMICS AND CHANGES OF MURMURS RESULTING FROM THEIR ACTION (TABLE V-VIII)

Digitalis

Digitalis increases the contractility of the heart and this is evidenced by an increase of rapidity and magnitude of left ventricular contraction. It decreases the automaticity of the heart and stimulates the vagus, thus prolonging ventricular diastoles and causing a slower rate. It increases cardiac output and decreases venous pressure, especially in patients with congestive failure.

In theory, the changes of cardiac dynamics caused by digitalis should result in an increase of all systolic murmurs, both in congenital and in acquired valvular diseases while diastolic murmurs would be variously affected. The full effect of digitalis on murmurs would be obtained after a few days of treatment unless large doses are administered intravenously.

A preliminary study was made in our laboratory using intravenous *ouabain*. Contrary to expectation, all murmurs arising in the left heart, whether aortic or mitral, systolic or diastolic, *decreased* after ouabain. This effect was only partly related to bradycardia and occurred even in patients with evidence of initial heart failure.

Amyl Nitrite

Amyl nitrite causes both systemic and pulmonary vasodilatation. It decreases arterial systemic pressure; it increases velocity of aortic flow and rapidity of left ventricular ejection; it increases the heart rate through a carotid sinus reflex. As a result, venous return to the right heart is increased within the first 15 to 30 sec. while that to the left heart is increased only after about 60 to 90 sec.

The pansystolic murmur of *organic mitral insufficiency* is decreased in the early phase by amyl nitrite. That of *"relative"* *mitral insufficiency* may either decrease or increase. The diastolic murmur of *organic mitral stenosis* is increased by amyl nitrite, largely on account of shorter diastoles causing higher left atrial pressure and more tumultuous flow through the mitral valve. In contrast, the murmurs caused by "relative" mitral stenosis (murmurs of C. Coombs, of A. Flint, of myocarditis, of left

ventricular failure) may decrease, due to decrease of left ventricular pressures. However, this change is not always found,
especially if there is left ventricular failure. Even the lack of
increase of the murmur during the phase of tachycardia caused
by amyl nitrite may be in favor of a functional diastolic rumble.
The systolic murmur of *valvular aortic stenosis* may either increase or decrease while that of *muscular subaortic stenosis* generally increases.

The action of this drug on murmurs of the right heart is of
particular interest. The blowing diastolic murmur of *pulmonary
insufficiency,* whether *organic or relative (G. Steell),* is usually
increased by amyl nitrite within the first 15 to 30 sec. due to
greater venous return and greater pulmonary flow. The harsh
ejection-type, systolic murmur of *pulmonary stenosis,* whether
organic or relative (pulmonary flow murmur including that of
some innocent murmurs), is also increased by amyl nitrite
through the same mechanism. The systolic murmur of *tricuspid
insufficiency* (organic or relative) and the diastolic murmur of
tricuspid stenosis (organic of relative) are generally increased
by amyl nitrite in an early period.

In regard to congenital shunts, here again amyl nitrite has
a significant diagnostic value. The systolic, ejection-type, pulmonary flow murmur of *atrial septal defect* is increased while the
pansystolic murmur of *ventricular septal defect* is decreased. In
ventricular septal defect with pulmonary hypertension, the murmur behaves like in any pulmonary flow murmur and therefore
increases. In *tetralogy of Fallot,* the murmur behaves as in ventricular septal defect, and therefore decreases. In regard to *patent
ductus,* the *uncomplicated form* shows a decrease of the murmur
while that *associated with pulmonary hypertension* may either
decrease or increase.

Methoxamine (Vasoxyl)

Methoxamine causes a constriction of the systemic resistance
vessels and an increase of left ventricular systolic pressure. Left
ventricular diastolic pressure is often also increased by large doses
of this drug. The rapidity of left ventricular contraction is
decreased.

The systolic murmur of *mitral insufficiency (organic or*

relative) is increased by the rise of left ventricular systolic pressure. The diastolic-presystolic murmur of *organic mitral stenosis* is decreased by the bradycardia that causes a lowering of left atrial pressures. On the contrary, that of *"relative" mitral stenosis* is increased by the left ventricular overload caused by methoxamine. In cases with atypical systolic murmurs, the murmur usually becomes more typical and easier to diagnose. The murmur of *valvular aortic stenosis* is decreased by methoxamine, and the same is true in *"relative" aortic stenosis (aortic flow murmur)*. The murmur of *muscular subaortic stenosis* is also decreased by methoxamine but to a greater extent because the increased resistance tends to decrease the gradient beteewn inflow and outflow tracts of the left ventricle.

The pulmonic systolic flow murmur of *atrial septal defect* increases in some cases. The pansystolic murmur of *ventricular septal defect* is constantly increased (increase of left ventricular pressure). An exception seems to occur when the ventricular septal defect is associated with pulmonary hypertension. In such cases, the murmur has been found to decrease by some authors.

The systolic murmur of *tetralogy of Fallot* is generally increased due to bilateral ventricular hypertension that increases the flow through the stenotic pulmonary valve.

The murmur of *patent ductus* is increased by methoxamine, except in cases with pulmonary hypertension, where either increase or decrease may be observed.

It is interesting to mention that, while in most cases of *pulmonary insufficiency* (whether organic or relative) the blowing diastolic murmur is not affected by methoxamine, a marked increase of the murmur has been noted in cases complicating the *Eisenmenger's syndrome*. In the latter, the increase of peripherel resistance causes an increase of pressure in both ventricles, an increased flow through the pulmonary valve, and an increased regurgitation.

Epinephrine (Adrenaline)

Epinephrine causes tachycardia, an increased rapidity of left ventricular contraction, and an increase of cardiac output. Even though it causes peripheral vasodilatation, cardiac output is so augmented that left ventricular and aortic systolic pressures are increased.

The changes caused by epinephrine are less typical than those caused by other drugs due to increase of both left ventricular energetics (similar to that caused by isoproterenol) and aortic pressure (similar to that caused by methoxamine). For this reason, epinephrine is not currently employed in our laboratory as a diagnostic test.

Norepinephrine (Nor-Adrenaline)

Norepinephrine has chiefly a peripheral effect causing constriction of both the resistance and the capacitance vessels. It is not usually employed as a diagnostic test but the changes caused by this drug would be similar to those caused by methoxamine.

Isoproterenol (Isuprel)

Isoproterenol increases the rapidity and power of contraction of the myocardium. It causes tachycardia, shorter systoles, and shorter diastoles. It causes dilatation of the systemic resistance vessels and also of the pulmonary vessels. Thus it causes greater flow, higher systolic pressure, and lower diastolic pressure in both the pulmonary artery and the aorta.

While isoproterenol increases the systolic murmur of *valvular aortic stenosis,* of *muscular aortic stenosis,* and of *"relative" aortic stenosis (aortic flow murmur),* the increase is greatest in muscular stenosis. For this reason, the use of this drug has diagnostic value for the clinical recognition of this form of obstruction. A similar behavior is encountered on the right side because the systolic murmur of *muscular subpulmonic stenosis* is enhanced much more than that of valvular or "relative" stenosis.

ROUTINE USE

One or more of the following drug tests should be used in cases with significant murmurs (Grade III and IV).

Vasodepressor Test with Amyl Nitrite by Inhalation

A control strip is recorded at a speed of 50 mm/sec. with the microphone over the best location of the murmur and suitable amplification. An electrocardiogram, phonocardiogram, and a tracing of the digital pulse are simultaneously recorded. The procedure should be explained to the patient, informing him of the transient nature of the response and of the particular smell of the drug. The patient should inhale deeply while the doctor breaks open the ampule. The physician should wait until a distinct increase in heart rate is noted (usually an increase of 15 to 30 beats per minute) and then take new records at the same speed and amplification until the pulse has returned to normal. A period of 10 minutes or more should elapse before proceeding with the vasopressor test.

Systemic Vasopressor Test with Methoxamine (Vasoxyl)*

A control pulse and blood pressure reading is taken. The procedure is explained to the patient. A control strip is recorded and an ECG and digital pulse tracing are taken. A dose of 5 mg of methoxamine (Vasoxyl) is diluted in 20 ml of 5 per cent dextrose and is slowly injected intravenously, 5 ml at a time, until the desired response is obtained.** Pulse and blood pressure are checked after each dose. The dose of 10 ml (2.5 mg) should not be exceeded in children less than 15 years of age. Once the response is obtained, repeated records are taken. The patient may be sent to the floor after this period with a brief note on the chart. An outpatient should be asked to wait for 60 minutes.

TABLE V—EFFECT OF DRUGS IN CONDITIONS CAUSING MURMURS IN THE LEFT HEART

Condition	Type of Murmur	Digitalis	Amyl Nitrite (Late Effect)	Methoxamine	Isoproterenol
Mitral insufficiency (organic)	Pansystolic	+ —	—	+	
Mitral stenosis (organic)	Diastolic-presystolic	—	+	—	....
Mitral stenosis (relative)	Diastolic-presystolic	—	—	+	
Aortic insuffciency	Early-diastolic	+ —	—	+	
Aortic stenosis (valvular)	Systolic, ejection type	+	+ —	—	+
Aortic stenosis (muscular)	Systolic, ejection type	+ +	+ + +	— —	+ + +
Aortic stenosis (relative)	Systolic, ejection type	+	+	—	+

*This test should *not* be performed in either children less than 5 years of age or hypertensive patients.

**Desired response consists of a rise in mean blood pressure by more than 10 mm Hg. This is accompanied by reflex bradycardia.

This test should be performed in patients with a systolic murmur over the left or right ventricular area.

Premature beats sometimes follow the use of methoxamine.

Myocardial Stimulant Test with Isoproterenol (Isuprel)

A control tracing is taken as described previously. The patient is instructed to place a table of isoproterenol (10 mg.) under his tongue. The tracing is then recorded on observing tachycardia or premature beat.*

TABLE VI—EFFECT OF DRUGS IN CONDITIONS CAUSING MURMURS IN THE RIGHT HEART

Condition	Type of Murmur	Digitalis	Amyl Nitrite (Early)	Isoproterenol
Pulmonary insufficiency (organic)	Early-diastolic	+	+	
Pulmonary insufficiency (relative)	Early-diastolic	—	+	
Pulmonary stenosis (valvular)	Systolic, ejection type	+	+	+
Pulmonary stenosis (muscular)	Systolic, ejection type	+ +	+	+ + +
Pulmonary stenosis (relative)	Systolic, ejection type	+	+	+
Tricuspid insufficiency (organic)	Pansystolic	+	+	+
Tricuspid insufficiency (relative)	Pansystolic	—	+ —	+
Tricuspid stenosis (organic)	Diastolic-presystolic	—	+	
Tricuspid stenosis (relative)	Diastolic-presystolic	—	+	

TABLE VII—EFFECT OF DRUGS IN CONGENITAL SHUNTS

Condition	Type of Murmur	Digitalis	Amyl Nitrite (Late Effect)	Methoxamine	Isoproterenol
Atrial septal defect	Systolic, ejection type		+ +	+ —	+
Ventricular septal defect	Pansystolic	+	—	+ +	+
Ventricular septal defect with pulmonary hypertension	Pansystolic or ejection type	—	+	—	+
Tetralogy of Fallot	Systolic	+	—	+ +	+
Patent ductus arteriosus	Continuous	+	—	+	+
Patent ductus with pulmonary hypertension	Systolic	—	+ —	+ —	+

After the test, the patient is asked to emit the tablet. The patient should be observed for 15 minutes after the test.

If no reaction is observed, the tracing should be repeated after intravenous injection of 0.02 mg of isoproterenol diluted in 10 ml of saline or dextrose solution.

This test should be performed in patients suspected of having muscular subaortic or pulmonary stenosis.

Vasopressor and isoproterenol tests should be performed at least 3 hours apart or on separate days.

Differential Diagnosis (Table VIII)

Certain diagnostic possibilities are not aided by the use of drugs. Thus, the pansystolic murmur of ventricular septal defect is affected in the same way as that of mitral insufficiency and that of the tetralogy of Fallot.

The following differential diagnoses, on the other hand, are currently aided by drug tests.

1. *Organic mitral stenosis versus relative mitral stenosis.* The diastolic rumble is *increased* by amyl nitrite in the organic stenosis; it may *decrease* (or at least fail to increase) in relative stenosis (Austin Flint and other functional diastolic murmurs). Methoxamine *decreases* the murmur of organic stenosis, often *increases* that of relative stenosis.

2. *Mitral stenosis versus aortic insufficiency.* The diastolic murmur is *increased* by amyl nitrite in mitral stenosis, *decreased* in aortic insufficiency. On the contrary, methoxamine *decreases* the murmur of mitral stenosis while it increases that of *aortic insufficiency.*

3. *Aortic insufficiency versus pulmonary insufficiency.* The diastolic murmur is *decreased* by amyl nitrite in aortic insufficiency, *increased* in pulmonary insufficiency. Methoxamine *increases* the murmur of aortic insufficiency, does not change that of pulmonary insufficiency.

4. *Pulmonary stenosis versus ventricular septal defect or tetralogy of Fallot.* Amyl nitrite *increases* the murmur of pulmonary stenosis, decreases that of the other two conditions. Methoxamine *increases* the murmur of ventricular septal defect as well as that of the tetralogy.

TABLE VIII—DIFFERENTIAL DIAGNOSIS BY MEANS OF DRUGS

	Mitral Stenosis (Organic)	Mitral Stenosis (Relative)	Mitral Stenosis (Organic)	Aortic Insufficiency	Aortic Insufficiency	Pulmonary Insufficiency	Pulmonary Stenosis	Ventricular Septal Defect	Tetralogy of Fallot	Valvular Pulmonary or Aortic Stenosis	Muscular Pulmonary or Aortic Stenosis
Amyl nitrite	+	−	+	−	−	+	+	−	−		
Methoxamine	−	+	−	+	+	+	−	+	+		
Isoproterenol										+	+++

5. *Aortic or pulmonary muscular stenosis versus aortic or pulmonary valvular stenosis.* The murmur is *increased* by isoproterenol in all these forms of stenosis; however, the increase is much greater in the muscular than in the valvular form. A similar result is obtained with ouabain.

6. *Organic versus relative pulmonary insufficiency.* In organic pulmonary insufficiency, ouabain causes an *increase* of the murmur by augmenting the power of right ventricular contraction, digitalis often *decreases* the murmur. This is particularly true of the relative pulmonary insufficiency caused by left heart obstruction (mitral stenosis) or left heart failure (decrease of left atrial and pulmonary pressures). It may not occur if the insufficiency is caused by pulmonary heart disease because the pulmonary pressure is less affected. Methoxamine *increases* the murmur of pulmonary insufficiency only in Eisenmanger's syndrome while it does not change that of other forms, whether caused by organic or relative insufficiency.

Chapter 23

Auxiliary Tracings

CAROTID TRACING

THIS TRACING is of value in the study of defects of the aortic valve, subaortic or supraaortic stenosis, coarctation, systemic hypertension or aortic aneurysms. It is also of value for the identification of the aortic component of the second sound and of an aortic ejection sound.

The tracing is recorded by applying a small funnel over the right carotid* or subclavian artery with a moderate pressure. The funnel is connected by short semi-rigid tubing to a piezoelectric transducer sensitive to low frequency vibrations, like that supplied by the Sanborn Company for pulse recordings. The transducer in turn is connected to an AC amplifier.

The normal carotid tracing presents a small wave during the tension period; a rapid rise, the onset of which coincides with either the *c* component of the first sound or an aortic ejection sound; a rounded or flattish top; a sharp drop, the trough of which (incisura) coincides with the aortic component of the second sound; a second wave (dicrotic wave) ; and several small subsequent oscillation. The normal tracing may show a minor indentation during the rise (or anacrotic slope), called anacrotic

---

*If recorded on the carotid artery, the funnel should be applied as low as possible. High carotid tracings already have a delay in the onset of rise and in the timing of the incisura.

depression. This, however, becomes much more marked in aortic stenosis (Fig. 51).

JUGULAR TRACING

The jugular tracing is of interest in lesions of the tricuspid valve, pulmonary heart disease, and congenital heart disease.

The jugular tracing is recorded with the same transducer and amplifier but the tube of the transducer is connected with the central opening of a pick-up provided with a double rim and a suction device.

The pick-up is applied over the right jugular bulb and fastened to the skin by suction. Then, the correct amplification is obtained, so that the various waves are clearly visible. If respiratory drift of the baseline is too wide, the tracing will be recorded in apnea.

The jugular tracing presents three positive waves and three negative waves. The positive waves are: *A,* coinciding with the presystolic contraction of the right atrium; *C,* coinciding with the early-systolic rise of the tricuspid valve and also with the early phase of the arterial pulse;* and *V,* coinciding with the opening of the tricuspid valve and the onset of ventricular filling. The negative waves are called Z (between *A* and *C*); X (between *C* and *V*); and Y (between *V* and *A*). The significance and alterations of these waves have been described in *A Primer of Cardiac Diagnosis* by myself and Sainani (1968) (Fig. 51).

HEPATIC TRACING

The interest of this tracing is similar to that of the jugular tracing. It is often more sensitive than the former and has the advantage that the *C* wave is not caused by arterial impact. This tracing is obtained by applying with marked pressure a large funnel to the right hypochondrium. The transducer and amplifier are the same as for the jugular tracing. The number and names of the waves are the same.

RESPIRATORY TRACING

This tracing is useful for interpretation of the respiratory

---

*The two phenomena may be dissociated, so that the *C* wave may become double, a first peak being caused by the valvular motion, a second peak being caused by the arterial impact.

variations of the second sound and of the respiratory variations of cardiac or vascular murmurs.

The method for recording respiratory tracings has been outlined in Chapter 22.

CARDIOGRAM

Various methods have been used for recording the ultra-low frequency movements of the precordium. These tracings record either displacement (Luisada, Johnston and Overy, Eddleman, Mounsey, Dimond and Benchimol) or acceleration forces (Rosa). The former authors have used a crystal microphone with a linear response, connected to the amplifier of an electrocardiograph.

The cardiogram can be recorded over any area of the precordium, and in any decubitus. That of the apex has been called the *apex cardiogram* (or apexcardiogram, or kinetocardiogram at apex) and is of interest for the study of the left heart. That recorded at the epigastrium is called *epigastric cardiogram* and is of interest for the study of the right heart.

The cardiogram is the resultant of several factors:

1. *Motions* of the heart and closer contact of the heart with the chest wall due to rotation of the apex and stiffening of the ventricular mass during systole.
2. *Volume* changes of the heart (decrease of the ventricular mass during ejection; increase during diastole).
3. *Pulsations* of the large arteries, indirectly transmitted.

Torsion of the heart and stiffening of the ventricular wall give rise to a closer contact of the apex with the chest wall. The cardiogram, recorded over the apex with the patient in sitting position or lying on his left side, is largely a tracing of motion. Emptying of the heart into the large arteries causes a reduction in ventricular volume which can be studied in animals by enclosing the heart in a cardiometer. The cardiogram obtained in man in the supine position near, but not over, the apex, is largely a volume tracing and resembles the experimental tracings. It frequently shows a drop of the curve during ejection. The various phases of ventricular filling during diastole are well recorded in any position but are best observed when the patient is lying supine. Arterial pulsations have only secondary importance in the apical cardiogram of normal hearts. However, the pulsation of a dilated aorta can modify the tracing to a great extent. When a cardiogram is recorded near the base of the heart, arterial pulsations and vibrations following the opening and closure of the semilunar valves are well recorded. The soft cushion formed by the lungs is often interposed between the heart and the chest wall reducing the amplitude of all waves, especially in inspiration.

The following description was advocated by me since 1953 (Fig. 51).

A small upright and rounded wave *(wave IV)* can be observed in the cardiogram during presystole. This is related to atrial contraction and is caused by the rapid flow of blood which enters the ventricles in this phase, as shown by cases of complete A-V block. It coincides with the IV sound (if this is present), hence its name.

The curve begins to rise at the beginning of ventricular systole *(notch IA)*. This rise starts between Q and R or at the peak of the electrocardiogram, and is synchronous with the first slow wave of the phonocardiogram in cases of atrial fibrillation. This rise is due to hardening of the ventricular mass during the tension period; its peak is simultaneaus with the first component of the I sound, i.e., the one that follows the closure of the mitral valve. A subsequent notch closely follows the opening of the aortic valve and the beginning of ejection into the aorta (notch IB). Then, the curve may rise further during the rise of the carotid pulse and may reach a peak that has been called *E* by others.

There may be two important variations from this scheme. In some cases, a positive plateau is present during systole (especially in the left decubitus). In others, a deep inverted wave may occur during ejection, changes of volume having predominance over effect of motion. The curve rises again after the systolic depression and reaches a peak soon after closure of the semilunar valves *(point II)*. This coincides with the aortic component of the II sound. From this point on, the various types of tracings become similar. The deepest trough is called *point O* and coincides with or closely follows the opening of the mitral valve. Its name is due to the fact that it is the lowest point of the tracing. Since diastole is accompanied by two phases of rapid inflow, there are two main diastolic waves in the cardiogram. The first is represented by the wave of rapid filling during early diastole. This is usually well defined and its peak is simultaneous with the III sound *(point III or RF)*. In exceptional cases, the polarity of all diastolic waves is inverted. Then the point *O* is positive and the point II is negative. After a few small undulations, a second phase of rapid filling, caused by atrial contraction, is marked by the small wave IV, as described above.

The cardiogram can be recorded in the various precordial sites that correspond to the electrode placements for the chest leads (V_1 to V_5) (Eddleman). Important data are revealed by comparing the various tracings.

TIMING OF CARDIAC EVENTS

The apex cardiograms have been used by various investigators to time certain heart sounds. An opening snap may be easily identified by its relationship to the onset of the ventricular filling movement (point *O*). This identification is less certain in some cases because a delayed pulmonary component of the II sound (IIP) also may coincide with the point *O*. A protodiastolic gallop, as well as a physiologic III sound, may be identified by their occurrence near the peak of the filling movement (point III). An atrial (or presystolic) gallop occurs close to the peak of the atrial wave (point IV).

Chapter 24

Interpretation of the Tracing

ONCE THE TRACING is recorded and mounted, interpretation should be done. This proceeds as follows.

1. *First Sound.* This is located by noticing that its beginning follows the QR wave of the electrocardiogram and precedes the rise of the carotid pulse. Its components are studied particularly at the midprecordium in the medium frequency bands. If there is an aortic ejection sound, it coincides with the rise of the carotid pulse. Splitting of the first sound (whether close or wide) is noticed and recorded.

2. *Second Sound.* This is located by noticing that its beginning coincides grossly with the end of the T wave of the electrocardiogram. Its components are well studied at the midprecordium and left base, especially in the medium and high frequency bands. The acceleration tracing is often excellent for this study. The aortic component coincides with the incisura of the carotid pulse; the pulmonary component normally follows. Inspiration usually widens the interval between the two components. However, a reversal of this sequence and of this dynamic behavior may occur and should be recorded.

3. *The Third and Fourth Sounds.* These are studied at the apex (left-sided) and at the midprecordium or epi-

gastrium (right-sided). The third sound coincides with the positive peak of rapid filling (wave III) of the apex cardiogram; the fourth sound precedes the Q wave of the electrocardiogram.

4. *The Opening Snap.* This is studied over all areas. It coincides with the deepest trough (point *O*) of the apex cardiogram.

5. *A Midsystolic or Late-systolic Click.* This usually has no electric or mechanical coincidence but precedes the second sound.

6. *Variations in Amplitude* of the heart sounds related to arrhythmias or respiration will be noted.

7. *Murmurs.* Murmurs are represented by long series of vibrations. One should note (a) their gross *position* in regard to sounds (systolic, diastolic, presystolic, continuous) ; (b) their predominant *frequency* (low-pitched, high-pitched), revealed by the filter necessary for their best recording; (c) their *shape* (diamond shape, crescendo, decrescendo, pansystolic, etc.) ; (d) their changes in relation to respiration* and to drug actions (see also Chap. 22).

Correlation between the deflections of the phonocardiogram and those of other auxiliary tracings is shown in Figure 51.

---

*According to Levin *et al.*, most murmurs decrease on *inspiration* when recorded on the surface of the chest. A greater number increase on inspiration if recorded within the right heart. Murmurs caused by tricuspid lesions increase on inspiration both within the heart and on the surface of the chest. According to these authors, respiratory changes are unreliable for their recognition except for tricuspid murmurs.

Chapter 25

Report

A PHONOCARDIOGRAPHIC report should give both a description of the findings and their interpretation. The latter can be done only after consideration of history, physical data, and electrocardiographic and roentgenological findings.

A sample of forms used for the report is presented below.

GRAPHIC REPORT

Xray findings_____   Date_____
_____   Referred by _____
                                         Performed by _____
Name_____Age_____Sex_____Clinic/Hosp. #_____Room_____
Auscultatory findings: _____
_____

Phonocardiogram
   First sound: _____
   Second sound: _____
   Systolic sounds: _____
   Diastolic sounds: _____
   Systolic murmurs: _____
                       _____
   Diastolic murmurs: _____
                       _____
   Continuous murmurs: _____
Precordial Cardiogram: _____
Arterial or Venous Pulse: _____
*Effect of Drugs or Respiration:*_____
_____

Interpretation: _____
_____
_____

Chapter 26

Artifacts

ARTIFACTS of the tracing can be easily recognized because the *vibrations* of the artifact do not occur for each cardiac cycle.

Extraneous occasional noises may be caused by crying, snoring or puffing of the patient; by sibilant, musical rales or by ronchi; or may be caused by rubbing of the chest piece against hair. The prolonged noise that accompanies inspiration causes a prolonged series of vibrations that are superimposed on the cardiac sounds.

An exceptional cardiac murmur, that tremendously increases from time to time, is the *systolic whoop*. This is an intrecardiac murmur that should be differentiated from extraneous noises.

Of course, *ambient noises* are recorded in the phonocardiogram if the proper conditions are not observed. In such cases, only short fragments of the tracing, or noise, at all, are suitable for interpretation.

Part VII

THE NORMAL VIBRATORY PHENOMENON OF THE PRECORDIUM

Chapter 27

Heart Sounds

THE DISPLACEMENT of the chest wall of the precordial area represents a periodic complex wave of definite configuration and magnitude for a person in basal conditions (Kountz *et al.,* Smith *et al.,* 1941 and 1941A, Foulger *et al.,* Johnston and Overy, Luisada and Magri, Eddleman *et al.,* Rosa). This periodic wave form reflects the complex vibratory phenomenon caused by the dynamic action of the heart and the effects it has on the large vessels. As such, it represents the additive result of a number of pure sinusoidal waves of different amplitudes and frequencies.

No matter how complex a wave is, it can be separated by means of Fourier's analysis into a number of sinusoidal components comprising the harmonics and overtones of the fundamental frequency (Goldman; McKusick *et al.,* 1954; Rodbard *et al.;* Geckeler *et al.*).

The periodic, complex wave of *displacement* of the chest wall constitutes a single physical entity whose energy content is equivalent to the total energy appearing across the chest wall. However, one can record a tracing of *velocity* (first derivative or rate of change of displacement) or of *acceleration* (second derivative or rate of change of velocity, or rate of rate of change of displacement). Thus displacement, velocity, and acceleration are three physical aspects of the same phenomenon. All three aspects of the vibratory phenomenon are currently recorded in our laboratory. Of course, low-frequency waves (like those of the normal III sound) are best recorded by the displacement tracing while high-frequency waves (like those of the II sound) are best recorded by a velocity or acceleration tracing.

The *spectrum of vibrations,* generated by the heart beat and transmitted through the tissues to the body surface, extends from a fraction of 1 cycle per second (1 hertz) to about 800 hz in the normal heart, and to 1,500 hz or more in certain cases with heart disease causing the appearance of soft, blowing murmurs. It overlaps only partly the auditory perception area (Fig. 4). A subdivision of the spectrum into *auditory* and *nonauditory* bands is, therefore, imposed by the limitations of the auditory system of man and not by a physical difference in the phenomenon under consideration.

PHYSICAL AND PHYSIOLOGIC ASPECTS OF THE FREQUENCY SPECTRUM

As the lower limit of auditory perception is generally about 20 hz (Chapter 5), this frequency can be considered as the dividing point separating the spectrum into an infrasonic band and an auditory (or sonic) band (Fletcher) (Fig. 4). The frequency components of the auditory band can be further subdivided into two adjacent bands (Zalter *et al.,* 1959):

1. A first band *(lower subliminal band)* extends from 20 hz to about 40 hz and is composed of vibrations of great magnitude. The energy level of these components, however, is not high enough to compensate for the low sensitivity of the human ear in this range. This band is, therefore, either inaudible or barely audible according to the intensity of the vibrations and the individual threshold of the observer.

2. A second band extends from 40 to 400 hz* and includes vibrations of gradually decreasing magnitude. As the ear is highly sensitive in this wide band, these vibrations are well perceived and constitute the most important section of the auditory band.

---

*With adequate amplification, vibrations of cardiac origin can be recorded above 400 cps. Their audibility is limited, however, so that for practical purposes a limit of 400 hz is more realistic than that of 1,000 hz previously suggested.

3. In the range above 400 hz the ear is still well able to perceive vibrations (its upper limit lies between 12,000 and 14,000 hz in adults). Because of a decline in amplitude, however, the vibrations of greater frequency have a proportionally smaller magnitude. Therefore, vibrations above 400 hz may be poorly audible or inaudible, not because of their high frequency but because of poor intensity. This band should be called the *upper subliminal band.*

Of the total vibratory spectrum, therefore, only the central band (40 to 400 hz) lends itself to good auditory perception (Fig. 4).

Another important factor to consider is that a progressive linear distortion is introduced by the auditory system because sensitivity for higher frequencies increases so as to approximately compensate for the smaller magnitude of the latter. Vibrations of higher frequency are heard as louder vibrations; therefore, any objective and correct analysis and evaluation of the audible part of the spectrum is impossible by the unaided ear, a fact that explains many current errors of auscultation.

The nature of the infrasonic vibrations has been the object of numerous studies and observations (Eddleman *et al.,* Johnston and Overy, Luisade and Magri, Rosa). Three superimposed patterns of motion are inscribed over the chest wall.

1. A total motion of the body, or *ballistic motion* of the thorax, falls in the ultralow- and low-frequency ranges (between 0 and 30 + hz).

2. A *local vibratory motion* of the chest wall relative to the rest of the thorax extends from the aforementioned frequency ranges to higher frequencies.

3. *Harmonics* and *overtones* from the other two motions may contribute to the spectrum of vibrations.

The infrasonic band includes, besides the *fundamental frequency,*[*] those *harmonics*[**] and *overtones*[***] that form the lowermost frequency components of the spectrum.

---

[*]*Fundamental frequency* is the lowest component frequency of a periodic quantity. It is equal to the inverse duration of the periodic pattern of the wave form. Thus, for a linear phonocardiogram (apex cardiogram) with a period (time interval of one cycle) of 0.8 sec., the fundamental frequency is 1/0.8, or

INTENSITY LEVEL

A gross evaluation of the intensity level of the different bands has revealed a tendency to a decrease with increasing frequency (Maass and Wber, McKusick *et al.,* 1955A). A first cause for this decrease is a physical factor, which requires that, for a given pressure, the amplitude of a sinusoidal wave decreases proportionally to the inverse of the square of the frequency (the so-called law of the square), i.e., at the rate of 6 db per octave for constant velocity. However, actual observations with calibrated apparatus indicate a greater and not uniform decrease as a result of physiologic factors (Luisada *et al.,* 1963).

A new study has been made recently by the author with Sakai and Feigen with new calibrated equipment. The first heart sound is larger over the midprecordium in comparison with the apex in the frequency band 30 to 60 hz but may become smaller for higher frequencies (Fig. 36). Its maximal amplitude is at about 40. Its drop in amplitude with higher frequency is either faster or slower than the 12 db slope from 60 to 120 hz, then becomes slower than such slope.

In regard to the second sound, the maximal amplitude is again at about 30 or 40 hz. The IIA (aortic) component tends to peak at 130-150 hz without reaching the magnitude that it has at lower frequencies. Then it drops, first faster, and then slower than the 12 db slope (Fig. 36). The IIP (pulmonic) component has a peaking at 70-80 hz, then drops slower than the 12 db slope, so that it is much smaller than IIA at 450 hz, and may even have disappeared (Fig. 36).

Speculations about the cause of these results include the following possibilities.

1. There may be inherent properties of the cardiac and vascular walls that generate high-frequency vibrations

---

1.25 hz or 75 cycles per minute, which corresponds to the heart rate. This should be differentiated from the resonant frequency, which is of the order of several cycles, both for the heart and the chest wall.

**A *harmonic* is a frequency component that is an integral multiple of the fundamental.

***An *overtone* is a frequency component, higher than the fundamental, that is not necessarily an integral multiple of the latter.

relatively larger than indicated by the law of the square.

2. There may be poor transmission of high-frequency vibrations through the mediastinum and lungs.

3. There may be a resonance of the chest wall that increases high-frequency vibrations.

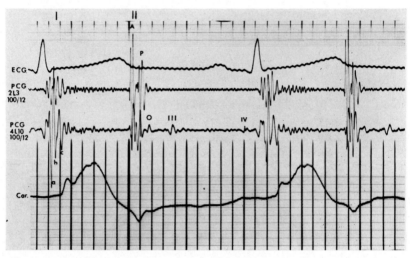

FIGURE 56. Phonocardiograms of a normal young individual recorded with modified Sanborn equipment. *From above:* ECG, phonocardiogram at medium frequency at the base; phonocardiogram at medium frequency at apex; apex cardiogram. Time = 40 msec.

The first factor may be investigated by intracardiac phonocardiography, a method that actually demonstrates a higher content of high-frequency vibrations than external phonocardiography. The second and third factors have been studied by Feigen *et al.*

It is interesting to note that all three properties may vary: the cardiac, because of cardiovascular disease; the pulmonary, because of pulmonary disease; and that of the thoracic cage, because of body build, sex, and age.

The precordial vibrations can be divided in various bands or sections of the total spectrum. Normal tracings in the various bands will be discussed now (Fig. 56-62).

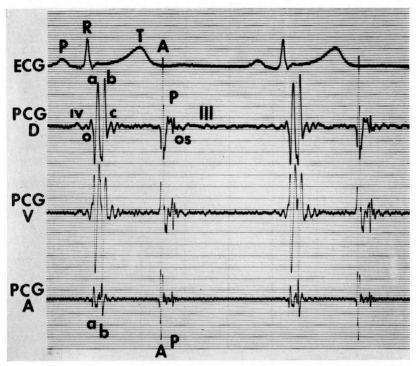

FIGURE 57. Phonocardiograms recorded at the apex in a young individual with General Electric equipment. *From above:* ECG, displacement, velocity, and acceleration phonocardiograms.

Band from 0 to 5 hz

The 0 to 5 hz band of vibrations corresponds to the visible and palpable motions of the chest wall (ultralow-frequency vibrations). It includes the apex beat, the epigastric beat, and several other motions of various intercostal spaces.

Following studies of Marey, Cushney, Hess, Weitz, Weber, Pachon, and others, it was studied by Luisada (1953), Luisada and Magri (apex cardiogram, epigastric tracing, and ultralowfrequency tracings of various intercostal spaces), Johnston and Overy (linear tracing), Eddleman (ultralow-frequency tracing or kinetocardiogram), Fishleder (1959), Benchimol *et al.* (1963), and Ueda *et al.* (1962A).

This band is subsonic because it is below the threshold of hearing.

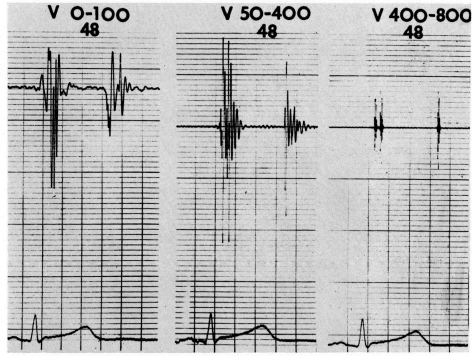

FIGURE 58. Velocity phonocardiograms recorded at the midprecordium in a normal, young individual with various degree of filtration with General Electric equipment.

Band from 5 to 30 hz

The band from 5 to 30 hz barely overlaps the audible range (Mannheimer, 1940; Rosa, 1948; Hollis; Dunn and Rahm, 1952; Schuetz; and Mounsey, 1959). This band is partly infrasonic (5 to 15 hz) and partly subliminal (15 to 30 hz); therefore, it is partly in that range where large vibrations may be perceived by the ear. An unfiltered phonocardiogram will give a fair tracing is the response of the microphone and amplifier is correct for this range. The best response is given by a displacement tracing; a velocity tracing is somewhat less accurate; and acceleration tracing is totally inadequate.

Band from 30 to 120 hz

The band from 30 to 120 hz was studied by Mannheimer. It was reproduced by the stethoscopic method of Rappaport and

Sprague (Sanborn Stetho-Cardiette). The most important octave band (60 to 120 hz) included in this wider band is well studied by the devices of Butterworth *et al.,* Maass and Weber, Holldack (t and m), Luisada and Zalter (1960) (30 to 60 hz), and Luisada and Bernstein (50 hz). This band is partly subliminal and partly auditory.

Band from 120 to 240 hz

The frequency band from 120 to 240 hz corresponds to the best area of recording of most apparatus and is well in the auditory range. This band was studied by Mannheimer, Maass and Weber, and Holldack (m^2); it corresponds to the low channel

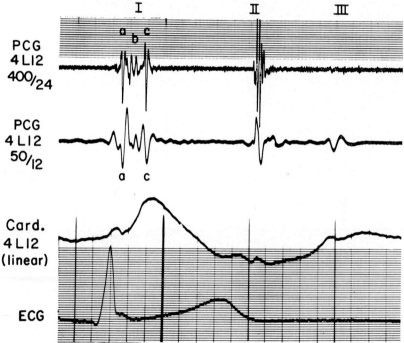

FIGURE 59. Phonocardiograms at apex and apex cardiogram recorded in a normal young individual with modified Sanborn equipment. Time = 40 msec.

of Leatham, to one of the channels of Butterworth, and to the third band of Luisada and Zalter (120 to 240 hz), as well as to the third band of Luisada and Bernstein (100 hz). The best response is obtained by using either a velocity or an acceleration tracing with a high pass filter at 100 or 120 hz.

Band from 240 to 500 hz

The frequency band from 240 to 500 hz corresponds to a good area of recording of many apparatus. It is approximately represented by the logarithmic method of Rappaport and Sprague. It corresponds to the middle channel of Leatham, to one channel of Butterworth, to one channel of Maass and Weber, as well as

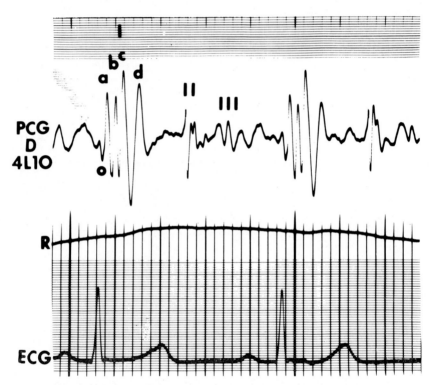

FIGURE 60. Displacement PCG without filtration recorded at the apex in a normal young woman with General Electric equipment. The four low frequency components of the first sound are visible.

Holldack (h[1]), to the fourth band (240 to 480 hz) of Luisada and Zalter, and to the fourth (200 hz) and fifth band (400 hz) of Luisada and Bernstein. It is well within the auditory range. Both velocity and acceleration tracings with high pass filter at 200-400 are adequate. However, if there is a sharp slope of filtration, we can record only tiny vibrations in this band.

Band from 500 to 1000 hz

The large band from 500 to 1000 hz corresponds already to that area of the spectrum where sounds originating in the heart and recorded from the chest wall are of extremely reduced magnitude. Audibility may be limited or even nil because of poor magnitude. Records have been taken in this band by Mannheimer, Maass and Weber, Holldack (h^2), Leatham, Luisada and Zalter (1960) (500 to 1000 hz), Luisada and Bernstein (600 hz). These high-frequency vibrations have been the object of a special study (Luisada and Di Bartolo), and are well recorded by photographing the screen of an oscilloscope. Equipment with a sharp slope of filtration seldom reveal vibrations in this band in normal subjects. They may reveal them in clinical cases.

Band from 1000 to 2000 hz

The band from 1000 to 2000 hz is usually subliminal because of the poor magnitude of the vibrations. Only few conventional apparatus, like that of Butterworth (full rotation) and the experimental apparatus of Luisada and Zalter (1960) are able to record vibrations in this band. The Japanese equipment modified by Ueda and Sakamoto* also seems capable of recording these high-frequency vibrations. Our new G.E. equipment is able to record them correctly. However, only rare clinical cases present murmurs in this band. The degree of amplification necessary for obtaining a significant tracing obviously increases from the low bands to the high bands. Certain apparatus (like the Elema and the standard Sanborn) have a preset degree of amplification, which automatically increases by a certain ratio when a higher band of frequency is selected. This ratio is based on the physical decrease of amplitude of higher frequencies, i.e., on a slope of 12 db per octave. Actually, the degree of amplification that is needed varies from subject to subject, and at times there is need of greater or lesser amplification for this band.

The Sound Vibrations of the Cardiac Cycle

The various phases of the cardiac cycle, identified by Frank, Wiggers, Schuetz, Holldack, Blumberger, and others will be now

---

*Personal communication.

reexamined on the basis of the data supplied by the various types of phonocardiograms.

PRESYSTOLE

Ultralow-frequency Tracing. A monophasic or diphasic wave (negative-positive) either at the apex or above the apex and at the epigastrium is revealed by this tracing (Luisada, 1953). It can be assumed that the first phase is caused by right atrial activity and the second by left atrial activity.

Low-frequency Tracing (5 to 30 hz). Two or three waves related to atrial activity during the P-Q interval of the ECG are revealed by the low-frequency tracing (Rosa, 1959, Mounsey, 1959). This is the IV sound of the heart.

Medium Low-Frequency Tracing. The phonocardiogram in the medium low-frequency range (30 to 60 hz) records the IV sound as a diphasic or triphasic slow wave (Luisada, 1953). Occasionally, three or four small vibrations can be recorded. It has been stated that this wave may fuse with the first sound and occur after the Q wave of the ECG (Schuetz *et al.*, Kincaid-Smith and Barlow, 1959). This is incorrect because the first sound itself starts with a slow vibration, which is present even in cases of atrial fibrillation (Luisada, 1953, Counihan *et al.*) or AV block (Schuetz *et al.*). On the other hand, children or adolescents with a short *P R* interval may have an atrial sound that continues with the first sound.

High-frequency Tracings. Occasionally, even normal subjects have one or two tiny vibrations in presystole which represent overtones of the IV sound.

VENTRICULAR SYSTOLE

This phase can be divided into *isovolumic* and *ejection periods* (Wiggers). More recently, another division was made (Schuetz, Holldack, Blumberger, and Fishleder), as follows:

1. The *electropressor latent period* is from the Q wave to the initial slow rise of (left) intraventricular pressure.
2. The *mechanoacoustic interval* is from the initial rise of (left) intraventricular pressure to the first group of rapid vibrations of the first sound; this was called *entrant phase* by Wiggers. Both 1 and 2 form the *electroacoustic interval* of Rosa.

3. The period of rapid rise of pressure continues beyond the opening of the aortic valve to about the peak of rapid ejection in the aorta. In the phonocardiogram, this period grossly corresponds to the period from the beginning of the first to the third main group of vibrations of the first sound (Luisada *et al.,* Shah *et al.*). There is a certain connection between this phonocardiographic interval and the isovolumic phase. However, the former is longer than the latter, which begins with mitzal valve closure and ends with aortic valve opening.

The phase of ejection was divided by Wiggers into *maximal ejection* (lasting until the peak of the aortic pressure curve) and *reduced ejection,* from this point to the onset of ventricular relaxation. *Protodiastole* lasts from the beginning of relaxation of the left ventricle to the incisura of the aortic pulse (Fig. 6).

Ultralow-frequency Tracing. The ultralow-frequency tracing with the pickup applied to the apex (apex cardiogram used by Luisada, 1953, Luisada and Magri, Rosa and Luisada, Benchimol *et al.,* 1963; kinetocardiogram used by Eddleman, 1962) often reveals two distinct waves, one during the entrant phase (mechanoacoustic interval) and another during the remaining course of rapid rise of pressure. The phase of ejection is often revealed by a systolic collapse caused by the reduced volume of the ventricular mass unless the apex maintains contact with the chest wall and causes a systolic plateau (more commonly found in the left decubitus). A combination of the two types (early rise, followed by descent) is common. End of systole is marked by a wave or notch (point IIa of Luisada, point K of Rosa and Luisada), which is usually positive but may be negative.

Medium Low-frequency tracing. The phonocardiogram in the medium low range (60 to 120 hz) * shows a small initial vibration of low frequency and magnitude during the mechanoacoustic interval (component O). It then shows a *Central phase of large vibrations* (Luisada *et al.,* 1949), which can often be subdivided into two or three main groups or components. The first two are 35-45 msec. apart; the third occurs from 60 to 70 msec. after the first and is usually smaller. In some cases, how-

---

*40-100 hz with high slope of filter.

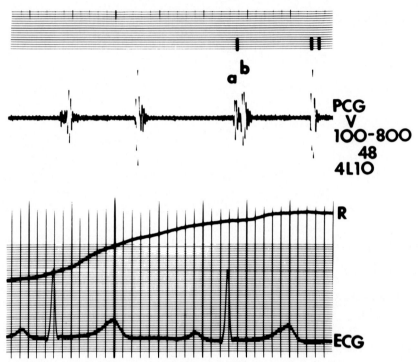

FIGURE 61. Velocity PCG with moderate filtration recorded at the apex in a normal young woman with General Electric equipment. The two high frequency components of the first sound are visible.

ever, the second group of vibrations is absent, and the third component is larger.

Subsequent to the opening of the aortic valve, the medium low-frequency tracing often presents from one to three vibrations in decrescendo that are connected with the early phase of ejection and terminate at the time of the peak of the aortic pulse. They seem to be caused by the vibrations of the aortic and pulmonic walls. The second half of systole is usually clear of vibrations.

In general, this band is the best for the study of the first heart sound. However, the second heart sound is also well recorded. In this band, both the aortic and the pulmonary components (if recorded over the 2nd-3rd left interspace) often have the same amplitude. The pulmonary component may be followed by a small vibration that corresponds to or closely follows in time the opening of the mitral valve.

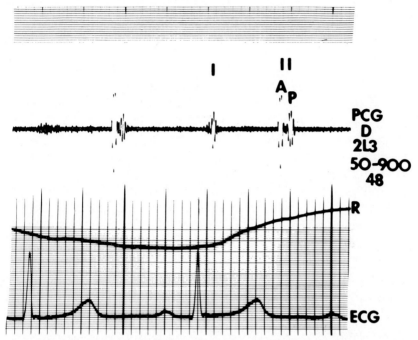

FIGURE 62. Displacement PCG with moderate filtration recorded over the second left space in a normal young woman with General Electric equipment. The two high frequency components of the second sound are visible.

Medium High-frequency Vibrations (Bands from 120 to 240 hz and 240 to 480 hz*). In the medium high-frequency bands, a common pattern occurs. The first sound often becomes split into two phases according to two possible occurrences. The first possibility (first shown by Leatham, 1956) is more commonly found in young individuals: the two groups of vibrations, separated by 35 to 45 msec., originate in the left ventricle (Luisada *et al.* 1961-1969). The largest may be either the first or the second *(close splitting)* (Fig. 57). The second possibility is more common in mature individuals. The two groups of vibrations, separated by 60 to 70 msec., originate in the left ventricle and the aorta, respectively *(wide splitting).* (Fig. 59). The second of these two groups of vibrations then corresponds to the third component of the first sound and could be called *ejection sound* in

---

*80-160 and 160-320 hz, respectively, with high slope of filter.

analogy with the term "ejection click" that has been used in clinical cases. It is caused by vibrations arising in the aorta during the first part of ejection.

These bands are also the best for the study of the second heart sound. This sound is made of two components that are more widely separated at the end of inspiration and are closer in expiration. The first of them is the aortic component (IIA), which is usually larger and of longer duration. The second is the *pulmonary component,* which is usually smaller and of shorter duration (Fig. 56).

*High Frequency Vibrations (Band from 500 to 1000 hz).**
High-frequency vibrations can be recorded in normal subjects only through great amplification and are particularly evident in young individuals with a thin and flat chest wall. Vibrations above 1000 hz are only exceptionally recorded, whereas those of an intermediate band (high pass at 600 hz or band pass at 600 to 1500 hz) can be studied in a larger number of individuals.

Due to its higher frequency, this band often records only the second heart sound. In this band, the aortic component of the second sound may show *two* groups of larger vibrations separated by about 15-20 msec. and followed by smaller aftervibrations. The pulmonary component of this sound is seldom recorded in this band.

ISOVOLUMIC RELAXATION PERIOD (IVRP)

The data supplied by the phonocardiogram are approximate because the IVRP begins with the beginning of ventricular relaxation, a point that can be determined only through catheterization, and ends with the mitral or tricuspid opening sound, which is only occasionally found in normal subjects.

IVRP of the left heart lasts approximately from the beginning of the aortic component of the second sound to the opening sound (or snap) of the mitral valve; IVRP of the right heart lasts from the beginning of the pulmonary component of the second sound to the opening sound or snap of the tricuspid valve.

Ultralow-frequency Tracing. A descending limb from the

---

*360-720 hz with high slope of filter.

peak IIa (closure of aortic valve) to the trough O (or IIb), which marks the lowest point of the tracing, is normally present in the ultralow-frequency tracing (Luisada, 1953). This point probably indicates tricuspid opening if the tracing is recorded at the epigastrium (in this area, there may be a mirror-like pattern with a low point at IIa and a peak at IIb), or mitral opening, if it is recorded at the apex and possibly also at the suprasternal notch (Luisada, 1953, Fishleder, 1959, Benchimol *et al.*).

Low-frequency (5 to 30 hz). In this band, certain subjects show a slow deflection marking the opening of the mitral valve. This is recorded best over the 3rd left interspace.

Medium Low-frequency Tracing (60 to 120 hz). The medium low-frequency tracing usually records 2 to 4 large vibrations that comprise the second heart sound. Frequently two larger components can be recognized within the central part of this sound *(aortic and pulmonary components)* as first shown by Leatham (1954).

Medium High-frequency Tracing (120 to 240 hz and 240 to 480 hz). In the medium high-frequency bands, two large vibrations usually emerge within the second heart sound in normal subjects. The best place for recording both vibrations is the third left interspace. Usually, only the first of them *(aortic component)* is transmitted to the second right interspace and toward the apex whereas the second *(pulmonary component)* is best transmitted to the 2nd and 1st left interspace. Occasionally, both components are well recorded at the 2nd right interspace. The two components of the second sound are well studied by comparing their changes during respiration. A sharp vibration corresponding to the mitral opening sound can be recorded in a few normal individuals, especially children, in the 3rd left interspace by using these bands (Luisada and Azgano).

High Frequency Tracing (500 to 1000 hz). If the high-frequency tracing is recorded at the base, usually the aortic component is revealed by a large vibration whereas the pulmonary component is revealed by either a tiny vibration or not at all.

DIASTOLE

Following Wiggers, diastole can be divided into rapid filling and slow filling (or diastasis).

Ultralow-frequency Tracing (0 to 5 hz). During diastole, the ultralow-frequency tracing rises from the lowest point (point O or IIb), to a high position (III), which marks the maximum of rapid filling and approximately coincides with the third sound. This part of the tracing is the most commonly reproducible and the most useful for identifying a third sound (Luisada, 1953).

Low-frequency Tracing (5 to 30 hz). A peak III represents the third heart sound and coincides with the peak of the phase of rapid filling.

Medium-frequency Tracing (60 to 120 hz). In the medium-frequency tracing, a small vibration may occur in coincidence with, or soon before, the peak of rapid filling *(third sound)*. It may be much larger in cases with increased filling of the left ventricle (triple rhythms or gallops) and it may be split (Luisada, 1952), thus simulating the occurrence of a fifth sound (Calo).

Medium High-frequency and High-frequency Vibrations (120 to 240 hz and higher). In normal subjects, no vibrations are recorded in diastole. In cases with pathologic triple rhythms, the *third sound* is usually recorded in the frequency band from 120 to 240 hz and, in certain cases, it may be recorded above 500 hz (Luisada and Di Bartolo).

The first and second sounds have a different content of frequencies at the apex and base. It is classic to admit that the first sound is larger at the apex and the second sound is larger at the base. This is usually not so as demonstrated by Sainani with the author; actually the first heart sound is usually largest over the midprecordium.

The relative amplitude of the heart sounds varies with the type of filter that is used. In the low and medium frequency bands, the first sound is as large as the second, especially over the midprecordium. In the high frequency bands, the first sound becomes small while the second increases in magnitude. In the very high frequency bands, the second sound is the only one recorded.

VALUE OF THE PHONOCARDIOGRAM IN VARIOUS FREQUENCY BANDS

Ultralow-frequency Tracing. The ultralow-frequency tracing is useful for identification of the first low vibration of ventricular systole; recognition of paradoxical movements of the ventricular wall (ventricular aneurysms, tricuspid insufficiency, some cases of constrictive pericarditis) and of right or left ventricular enlargement; recognition of a triple rhythm or of an opening snap of the mitral valve through coincidence of the various sounds with the waves of this tracing.

Low-frequency Tracing. The low-frequency tracing is useful for recognition of the first slow vibration that initiates ventricular systole; for recording the slow vibrations of the third or fourth sound or their summation; and for a study of the sound changes that take place in the course of valvular lesions, myocarditis, hypertension, and coronary heart disease.

Medium Low-frequency Tracing. An overall picture of the heart sounds and of the rumbling cardiac murmurs can be obtained through the medium low-frequency tracing. It clearly presents those vibrations of early systole that occur in conditions accompanied by an enlargement of the aorta or pulmonary artery; it reveals the third or fourth sound; it shows the opening snap of the mitral valve moderately well, and shows well the diastolic rumble of mitral stenosis.

Medium High-frequency Tracing. The medium high-frequency bands reveal the two high-pitched components of the first sound; most of the cardiac murmurs, particularly the presystolic murmur of mitral stenosis and the systolic murmurs of aortic and pulmonary stenosis, as well as the average early-diastolic murmur of aortic insufficiency; the opening snap of mitral stenosis; some of the high-pitched vibrations of triple rhythms (gallop rhythms) ; and the murmurs of VSD and PDA.

High-frequency Tracing. The high-frequency bands reveal best the blowing, high-pitched murmurs of mitral, tricuspid, or aortic insufficiency; the high-pitched aortic component of the second sound; the vibrations of systolic snaps and of friction rubs; the murmurs of VSD and PDS; and again the murmurs of aortic or pulmonary stenosis.

Chapter 28

Correlation Between Phonocardiographic Waves and Those of Other Tracings

Phonocardiogram and Tracing of Pressure (Fig. 6)

THE FIRST rapid component (comp. *a*) of the first sound falls during the first part of left ventricular (LV) pressure rise and during the rise of the first derivative of this pressure. The interval between onset of pressure rise and onset of this component averages 30 msec.

The second component (comp. *b*) occurs 30 to 40 msec. later and corresponds with onset of aortic pressure rise; it usually coincides with a notch of the first derivative of left ventricular pressure or with its peak.

The third component (comp. *c*) occurs 60 to 70 msec. after the first, at a time when the aortic pressure is reaching its first peak. Again, it coincides with a notch of the first derivative of LV pressure. An aortic ejection sound (a pathologic phenomenon) would occur 15 to 20 msec. later.

The aortic component of the second sound grossly coincides with the incisura of the aortic tracing and with the negative peak of the first derivative of LV pressure.

The pulmonary component of the second sound grossly coincides with the incisura of the pulmonary artery tracing.

The opening sound or snap of the mitral valve either coincides with the lowest point of the LV pressure tracing or follows it closely.

The third sound grossly coincides with the peak of rapid filling of the LV pressure tracing and with the return to the baseline of the first derivative of this pressure.

Phonocardiogram and Carotid Tracing

If the carotid tracing is recorded low in the neck, the relationship between sounds and carotid tracing is similar to that between sounds and aortic pressure tracing. Thus, the first two components of the first heart sound precede the rise of the carotid pulse while the aortic component of the second sound coincides with the incisura. If the tracing is recorded on a higher level in the neck, then the incisura follows the aortic component.

Phonocardiogram and Jugular Tracing

The *a* wave usually ends during the first sound. The *c* wave follows the first sound. The *v* wave follows the second sound. The peak of this wave occurs a short interval after the opening of the tricuspid valve but coincides or follows the opening of the mitral valve. It should be kept in mind that transmission of the volume wave from the heart to the neck causes some delay of this peak.

Phonocardiogram and Apex Cardiogram

A small wave of the apex cardiogram (ACG) may coincide with the fourth sound. The *o* component of the first sound coincides with the initial rise of the ACG. The first rapid component (comp. *a*) of the phonocardiogram coincides with the very first part of the rise of the ACG. The peak of the ACG may coincide with either the third component (comp. *c*) of the first sound or an ejection sound.

The aortic component of the second sound coincides with a small notch of the ACG.

The opening snap coincides with the lowest point of the ACG (point *O*).

The third sound coincides with the peak of the wave III of the ACG (wave of rapid filling).

Chapter 29

Duration of Sounds – Intervals – Amplitude

K NOWLEDGE OF THE DURATION of a sound is essential
for determination of sound abnormalities including prolongation of sounds and occurrence of short murmurs. The
intervals between components of sounds, as well as between sounds
are of great importance, both for interpretation of sounds and
for recognition of cardiovascular abnormalities. For these reasons,
numerous studies were devoted to the study of such measurements in the past. Unfortunately, such studies give different
figures according to the technical characteristics of the equipment used and also according to the criteria used in the
determination.

The duration of heart sounds was repeatedly investigated
by Luisada *et al.* (1949, 1963). The study of 1949 was made
with the Sanborn "stethoscopic system," and a similar study was
subsequently made with similar technique by Ongley *et al.*
(1960). In 1963, we repeated the study in 10 normal subjects
by using a specially-built calibrated system.

We have recently repeated again such study in 23 normal
young subjects by using the new General Electric calibrated
system. Due to the fact that displacement tracings are more
difficult to study on account of less sharp beginnings and ending of sounds, the study was made for velocity tracings with
different types of filtration and for unfiltered acceleration trac-

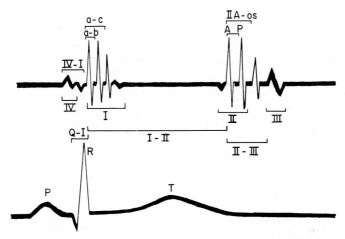

FIGURE 63. How to measure duration of sounds and their intervals.

ings (Aravanis *et al.*, 1970). In the measurements of duration, *the onset and ending of a sound* should be considered (Fig. 63). Statistical analysis of the data was made, and the following data were studied: the mean; the standard deviation (corrected for small samples); the standard error of the mean; the maximum and minimum values. All the minima and maxima were found to fall within the 98% limits. When less than 5 subjects presented a certain phenomenon, the figure was omitted. In Tables IX, X, XI, the figures from above are: mean value, minimum value, and maximum value.

Q-I Interval

A delay in the onset of the first sound in mitral stenosis was described by Weiss and Joachim and was confirmed by Cossio and Berconsky, as well as by many others. This is one of the reasons why measurement of this interval is important in clinical phonocardiography.

To decide whether or not the first sound is delayed, it is necessary to measure the Q-Ia interval, i.e., the interval from the onset of the Q wave of the electrocardiogram to the onset of the first component of the first heart sound. Obviously, agreement should be reached about the conditions of measurement. As far as the ECG is concerned, any lead showing a good Q wave will be adequate. In regard to the phonocardiogram, it should be kept in mind that some changes may be caused by the filter. If a medium-high filter is used, the first (low-frequency) group of vibrations will be abolished and the Q-I interval will become longer.

Sakamoto *et al.* (1960) found an average Q-I of 50 msec. in normal adults. Kelly studied this interval in 75 patients with mitral stenosis and 100 patients with other forms of heart disease (patients with QRS intervals longer than 0.11 sec. were excluded). They found an average Q-I interval of 40 msec. (± 10) in heart disease without mitral stenosis including 25 patients with mitral insufficiency. In mitral stenosis, the average interval was 60 msec. (± 30). None of the patients without mitral stenosis had an interval longer than 70 msec. whereas 45 per cent of those with mitral stenosis had an interval greater than 70 msec.

Messer *et al.* confirmed that the Q-I interval varies in atrial fibrillation with the length of the previous cycle, a fact previously described by me (1941). No such variation was found by Kelly in patients with atrial fibrillation unless they also had mitral stenosis.

Prolongation of the Q-I interval has been noticed by Ongley *et al.* (1960) in patients with congenital heart dicease. A prolongation was found also in arterial hypertension (particularly if there was aortic insufficiency) by Weissler *et al.*, Puchner *et al.* (1960A), and Sakamoto *et al.* (1960). The latter found an average Q-I interval of 64 msec. in hypertensive patients without heart failure and 77 msec. in hypertensive patients with heart failure. On the other hand, occasional cases of severe mitral stenosis with a normal Q-I interval do occur (Ongley *et al.*, 1960).

In our recent study, the Q-I interval was found longer over the base on account of lack of recording of some early sound vibrations. It was found longer in tracings recorded with high filtration for the same reason. Therefore, present day clinical comparison should be made only with the data pertaining to either the apex or the midprecordium, and excluding the tracings at 400-800 filtration. The average values were 55, 55, 59, msec. at the apex; 57, 57, 62 at the midprecordium according to filtration. The maximum values were 70, 75, 60, 65, for velocity tracings, and 80, 80 for acceleration tracings according to filtration. Therefore, if one uses a velocity tracing, prolongation of the Q-Ia interval can be stated only if the interval is *longer than 75 milliseconds* on account of occasional longer intervals of a few normal subjects. This is somewhat longer than the previously accepted value.

Ia-Ib Interval. This interval measures the distance between the two main high-frequency components of the first sound. It was found as long as 60 msec. (midprecordium, velocity 0-100), and as short as 10 msec. (apex, velocity 400-800). Its average was 32, 30 (apex); 33, 27 (midprecordium); with shorter intervals for high filtration (19, 20) or acceleration tracings (26, 25).

Ia-Ic Interval. This interval measures the distance between the first and third components of the first heart sound. Its prolongation should be considered as evidence that there is an "ejection sound" and therefore there is some cardiovascular abnormality. The average figures were 63, 58 (apex); 65, 56 (midprecordium); and 57, 52 (base) for velocity tracings; and 53, 52, 57 for acceleration tracings over the three areas. The longest interval found was 90 msec. for velocity tracings 50-100 at apex; intervals of 80 msec. were not unusual, however, with various filters and over the various areas. Thus, an interval of 80 or 90 msec. cannot be considered pathological in a clinical case on account of occasional longer intervals of a few normal subjects.

Q-II Interval

The Q-IIA and the Q-IIP segments of the Q-II interval can be used as simple determinable indices of the duration of systole for each ventricle.* Boyer and Chisholm studied the individual components of the second sound by employing the first sound as the reference point. They analyzed the I-IIA and I-IIP intervals (the distance from the first sound to the aortic component and

---

*Recent studies from our laboratory (Luisada and MacCanon, 1971) have shown that the Q-II interval may become considerably longer than the duration of systole, especially in aortic stenosis (delay of IIA) and atrial septal defect (delay of Q-IIP).

pulmonary component, respectively) during normal respiration, and described a dual mechanism for the inspiratory increase in the interval between the two components of the split second sound. Shafter repeated the study in 15 normal subjects and in patients with atrial septal defects. Castle and Jones investigated the respiratory variations in 68 normal children by measuring the interval from the peak of the R wave to the components of the second sound. Aygen and Braunwald presented studies of 51 normal subjects in whom they measured the Q-IIA and Q-IIP intervals, and evaluated the splitting of the second sound in atrial septal defect comparing the Q-IIP intervals of these patients with those of normal subjects.

The *Q-IIA Interval* (i.e., the interval from the onset of the Q wave to the onset of the aortic component of the second sound) includes the distance from the Q wave to the onset of left ventricular pressure rise plus the total duration of left ventricular systole (from the onset of pressure rise to the aortic incisura) .* It has been shown that, in the absence of conduction disturbances, the interval from the Q wave to the onset of left ventricular pressure rise is relatively constant. This suggested a constant relationship between the Q-IIA interval and total left ventricular systole.

Shah and Slodki plotted the averages of the Q-IIA intervals obtained in 18 normal, anesthetized dogs against the duration of left ventricular systoles measured in the same cycles. A high degree of correlation was evident. They also established rate-corrected, normal standards for Q-IIA and Q-IIP intervals in 112 normal subjects, thereby providing a reference standard for the second sound in the evaluation of disease states.

Aortic Component. The predicted Q-IIA interval for a given R-R interval can be expressed as:

$$Q\text{-}IIA = 61.6 + 10.24 \sqrt{R\text{-}R}$$

---

*It is assumed here that the aortic component of the second sound coincides with the aortic incisura, a fact that has been confirmed by Mori *et al.* However, closure of the aortic valve occurs somewhat earlier (MacCanon *et al.*) It should be kept in mind that end of systole is followed very soon (7-13 msec.) by semilunar valve closure in normal subjects. However, another short interval occurs between valve closure and component of the second sound (MacCanon *et al.*; Luisada and MacCanon) .

No significant effect of age on the Q-IIA interval was noted within the range studied (21 to 50 years of age), and no effect of the different normal blood pressure levels (systolic pressures between 105 and 140 mm. Hg were observed).

Pulmonary Component. A linear dependence of the end-expiratory Q-IIP interval on the square root of the R-R interval was again noted. A small but statistically significant linear dependence on age was also demonstrated and can be expressed as:

$$Q\text{-IIP} = 98.9 + 10.631 \sqrt{R\text{-}R} - 8.860 \text{ Age}$$

For each additional year of age, the Q-IIP interval decreases by 0.860 msec., thus resulting in a reduction of about 25.8 msec. in 30 years.*

Considering the importance of a safe method of determining left atrial pressure, several formulas have been studied based on the Q-I and IIA-os intervals. At their foundation resides the belief that, the higher the left atrial pressure, the longer will be the Q-I (delayed closure of mitral valve) and the shorter the II-A-os interval (earlier opening of the mitral valve).

The most reliable seems to be the formula dervised by Yigitabasi *et al.* (1969) *:

mean LA pressure = 17.8 [(Q-1) / (II-A-os)] : 1.33
(mm Hg)

However, it is likely that this formula will give the pressure gradient across the mitral valve and not the actual pressure. Still, if proven correct, it would be invaluable for clinical assessment of the severity of mitral stenosis.

Effect of Age. In end-expiratory apnea, no significant effect of age can be demonstrated on the aortic component, whereas the Q-IIP interval is statistically related to age. Splitting of the second sound greater than 20 msec. is rare in both phases of respiration in the age group from 41 to 50 years as compared to younger subjects. This emphasizes the need to consider the factor of age in the evaluation of the second sound in disease states.

---

*This dependency is based on data gathered from patients between the ages of 21 and 50. Extrapolation in either direction is not justified.

---

*Personal communication.

It is interesting to note that *advanced age* shows a different phenomenon, studied by Slodki *et al.* (1969). First, there is a prolongation of both Q-IIA and Q-IIP. This prolongation may be greater for the one or for the other, so that, out of 16 subjects between 70 and 92 years of age, normal splitting was found in 37% and reverse splitting in 25%, the rest (38%) having a single second sound.

Phonocardiographic studies in *newborn infants* (Craige and Harned) showed that splitting of the second sound is minimal (less than 20 msec.) in the first few hours of life and gradually increases to a maximum of 30 msec. between 48 and 165 hours. These variations are attributed to the hemodynamic changes occurring in the neonatal period.

With the exception of patients with severe pulmonary hypertension, the pulmonary component of the second sound has fewer high-frequency vibrations than the aortic component. Thus, when passing from a lower to a higher frequency band, the pulmonary component may be equal to the aortic up to 100 to 150 hz, becomes smaller than the aortic above 100 hz, and may disappear above 300 or 400 hz leaving only the aortic component.

IIA-IIP Interval. This interval measures the distance between the aortic and pulmonary components of the second sound. As longer intervals can be found in clinical cases, the interest centers around the longest intervals that are found in inspiration and especially those measured at the base. In our recent study over this area, the average intervals were 47, 43, 44, 45. The maximum intervals were 60, 50, 50, 55 according to the type of filter and the type of tracings. Thus, an interval of 60 msec. in inspiration cannot be considered abnormal in an adult.

INTERVAL BETWEEN THE SECOND SOUND AND THE OPENING SOUND OR SNAP (IIA-os)

The interval between the aortic component of the second sound and the mitral opening snap measures approximately the duration of the isovolumetric relaxation period. This phase, which can be measured by comparing simultaneous intracardiac and aortic pressure tracings, average about 40 msec. in a dog with a heart rate of 75 (Wiggers) * and was found in man in the range of 50 to 110 msec. by Braunwald *et al.* (1956).**

The duration of the isovolumic relaxation period has notable importance because, if it were possible to measure it by means of a nontraumatic procedure like phonocardiography, it would permit us to evaluate the level of pressure of the left atrium.

Since the report of Margolies and Wolferth, the interval between the aortic component of the second sound and the mitral snap was considered equivalent to the isovolumic relaxation period of the left heart, and a fairly close correlation was found between this interval and the level of the left atrial pressure measured on catheterization (Messer *et al.*, Mounsey, 1953, Wells, 1954, Kelly, Leo and Hultgren, Haring *et al.*, 1956, Dack *et al.*, Di Bartolo *et al.*, 1962). Patients with severe mitral stenosis have the shortest interval (50 msec.), whereas patients with mild mitral stenosis have the longest interval (120 to 130 msec.).

The average left ventricular relaxation period is 80 msec. and the maximum normal is 120 msec. (Arevalo and Sakamoto, 1964).

Clinical phonocardiography has shown that the interval between the aortic component of the second sound and the opening sound of the normal mitral valve ranges between 50 and 110 msec. with an average of 85* (Luisada *et al.*, 1964).

Intervals in Patients with Prosthetic Valves. The phonocardiograms of patients with prosthetic aortic or mitral valves have distinct opening and closing clicks, which have been used for measuring the various phases of cardiodynamics. It should be kept in mind that the obtained data are not accurate because (1) a residual degree of stenosis is constant, and (2) opening and closing of such valves requires higher pressures than in the case of normal valves (Shah *et al.* 1963A).

The IIA-os interval can be measured only in some normal

*In our laboratory, this interval measured an average of 60 msec.

**These measurements were made through open-chest procedures in three subjects submitted to thoracotomy.

*This study was made in 10 normal subjects (out of 35) having an opening sound (average 89 msec.) and on 6 subjects (out of 24) with minimal mitral insufficiency or stenosis having an opening sound (average 85 msec.).

individuals and thus it acquires particular interest. In our recent study, the average data were 75, 70 (apex); 73, 70, 69 (midprecordium); and 75, 70 (base).

The longest interval is of importance considering the occasional confusion between opening snap and third sound. It was found to be 90, 80 (apex); 80, 80, 80 (midprecordium); and 80, 80, 80 (base). Thus the *longest normal interval* is 90 msec., still much shorter than the shortest II-III interval (see below). It is still shorter than some intervals found in mild mitral stenosis or after commissurotomy, a fact that seems to point out additional elements that may prolong this interval in the above cases. The *shortest normal interval* was found to be 65, 65 (apex); 60, 55, 55 (midprecordium), 70, 60 (base). Thus, one can occasionally encounter intervals as short as those found in mitral stenosis. This indicates that the IIA-os interval alone is not sufficient for evaluation of left atrial pressure, as also confirmed by Yigitabasi *et al.* (see above).

The IIA-III Interval. The interest of this interval is based on the need for undeniable recognition of a third sound. In our study in young adults, the minimum value was 120 msec. and the maximum value, 160 msec., both at the apex. Thus, a wide margin separates the minimum value of this interval from the maximum value of the IIA-os interval and excludes the possibility of misinterpretation.

DURATION OF SOUNDS

Duration of I. Average duration is significant only in velocity tracing recorded at apex or midprecordium with low filtration due to predominance of low frequency vibrations ending this sound in displacement tracings. In our study, it was found to be 122 and 115 msec., respectively. The longest sound was 160 msec. at the apex (velocity 0-100). Thus, only if a first sound lasts longer than 160 msec., can one accept the fact that there is an early-systolic murmur.

Duration of II. The duration of the second sound obviously depends on the width of the A-P interval. However, it should be mentioned that the longest second sound was 60 msec. (base, inspiration, velocity 0-100). Thus, any longer sound would represent the beginning of an early-diastolic murmur or the addition of an extra-sound.

Duration of III. Usually, this sound lasts from 70 to 80 msec. However, shorter sounds (40-50 msec.) and longer sounds (100) were observed. In order to state that there is a pathological mid-diastolic murmur, one should observe a series of vibrations that is longer than 100 msec.

Duration of IV, duration of II. The duration of the fourth sound has less significance for clinical comparison and can be found in Tables IX-XI.

PHONOCARDIOGRAM OF THE INFANT

Normal newborn infants were studied by Craige and Harned. They found (1) an early systolic click appearing at birth but later diminishing in frequency and occurring an average of 39.7 msec. after the onset of the first sound; (2) a second systolic click, occurring an average of 63.9 msec. after the onset of the first sound; (3) a narrowly split second sound, which became more widely split later (the average was 19.4 msec.) at 6 to 8 hours of life; and (4) a transient, low-intensity systolic murmur in one-third of the patients. These data still need confirmation and interpretation.

PHONOCARDIOGRAM OF THE AGED

According to Aravanis and Harris, the average duration of the heart sounds is moderately prolonged in the aged; with increasing age, the total duration decreases while the central phase remains practically unchanged.

A fourth heart sound was found by Aravanis and Harris in 21 per cent of their patients, and by Bethel and Crow in over one-half of their patients. The third sound was rare in the Aravanis and Harris series but was found in more than one-fourth of the patients of Bethel and Crow. A large, low-pitched vibration was found at the end of the first sound (vascular vibration) in a large percentage of patients by Aravanis and Harris. No significant murmurs were found by Aravanis and Harris in contrast with Bethel and Crow, who found a systolic murmur (ejection in type) in nearly 60 per cent of their patients. The discrepancy between these two series is probably the result of more rigid criteria of selection of Aravanis and Harris, who excluded hypertensive patients and subjects with definite electrocardiographic abnormalities.

Chapter 30

The Heart Sounds of Mammalians

THE HEART SOUNDS of horses have been recorded first by Bressou, Neumann-Kleinpaul and Steffan, and Charton *et al.* My co-workers and I (1944) made a study of normal animals and a study of animals under the influence of various drugs. Many experimental studies have been made in dogs; therefore, the normal heart sounds of this animal are among the best known (Chap. 3). More recent studies of heart sounds in the horse were made by Corticelli and by Patterson *et al.;* studies in the monkey and in the cat were made by Hamlin *et al.;* studies in mice were made by Richards *et al.*

Recording Technique

The recording technique is identical to that used in humans. A microphone with a large bell should be used in large animals, whereas a small bell is preferable in small animals. It is placed to either the right or left of the sternum; it is held by means of a rubber strap in large animals while, in rabbits and smaller animals, it should be held by hand.

Phonocardiographic Data

The multiplicity of phonocardiographic data renders necessary its summarization (Tables XII, XIII). Table XII was made from older data obtained by means of a Sanborn Stethocardiette, while Table XIII was made from recent data obtained through use of our new General Electric setup in selected specimens of various species.

Representative tracings are presented in Figures 64 to 70.

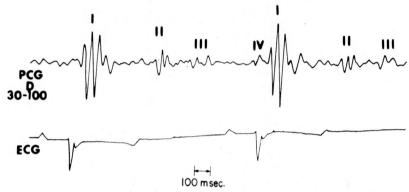

FIGURE 64. Electro- and phonocardiogram of a pony. Displacement tracing 30-100 Hz. A double third sound and a fourth sound are visible in diastole.

Heart Rate. This rate increases from the larger to the smaller animals, though without an exact correlation with the weight of the heart. The most striking evidence of this is the minor increase in rate between guinea pig and white mouse in spite of a nearly 1:175 ratio in heart weight.

Q-I Interval. This interval becomes shorter with decrease in heart size but again without an exact correlation. The Q-I interval of the white mouse (the shortest) is about one-third that of man. As this interval measures the electric activation of the

TABLE XII—OLDER DATA CONCERNING PHONOCARDIOGRAMS IN ANIMALS

Species	Fourth Sound	First Sound (msec.)	Second Sound	I-II	Third Sound
Bull	+	120-200	40-60	320	—
Cow	—	120-200		520	—
Horse	+	150-240	80-100	520-620	+
Pony	+	120	80-100	600	+
Donkey	—	140-160	70-120	440-580	+
Pig	+	120-200	40-60	280	—
Sheep	—	70	40-60	280	—
Goat	—	70	60	280	—
Small monkey	+	60-95	35-40		—
Dog	—	80	60	200-240	+
Cat	—	50	40	180	—
Rabbit	+	40	40	180	—
Guinea pig	+	30	20-30	120	—

These data are from Luisada *et al.* (1944) except for those of small monkeys (mulatta macaca), which are from Hamlin *et al.*

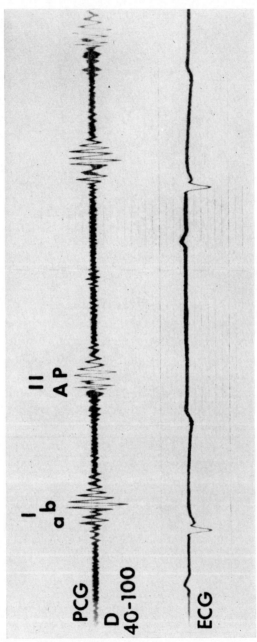

FIGURE 65. Electro- and phonocardiogram of a pony. Displacement tracing 40-100 Hz. The first sound shows the *a* and *b* components; the second sound shows the *A* and *P* components.

Table XIII—Data From Electrocardiograms and Phonocardiograms in Selected Individuals of Various Species

Species	Heart Weight (gm)	Electrocardiogram			Phonocardiogram					
		Rate per min.	P-Q (msec.)	Q-T (msec.)	Q-I (msec.)	No. Comp. of I	Interval Ia-Ib (msec.)	Duration of I (msec.)	No. Comp. of II	I-II
Pony	1600	50	200	460	50	3	65	150	2	500
Man	320	70	180	400	55	3	40	140	2	350
Dog (large)	130	90	100	280	50	3	30	100	2	204
Cat	18	160	70	230	30	3	13	40	2	190
Rabbit	10	240	60	130	20	3	12	30	1	120
Guinea pig	2.5	420	60	120	20	2	12	30	2	120
White rat	1	440	30	75	20	2	12	20	1	50
White mouse	0.15	480	25	50	18	2	12	15	1	50

septum and the ventricles plus the time for the initial increase of left ventricular pressure, this fact seems to indicate a less rapid spreading of the impulse and a similar development of ventricular tension in smaller animals.

Components of I. Either three or two main components were recorded in all species. Two components only were found in the guinea pig, rat, and mouse. However, it is likely that the third component, always small in normal subjects, may be easily missed in smaller animals.

Interval Between a and b Components of the First Sound. This interval decreases from the larger to the smaller animals. It is longer in the pony (65 msec.) than in man (40 msec.) and dog (30 msec.). In all smaller animals, it has about the same duration (12-13 msec.) in spite of a marked difference in heart size and heart rate from the cat to the white mouse.

Duration of the First Heart Sound. Taking the heaviest and the lightest heart, we note a 1:10 ratio in duration. This should be compared to a gross 1:100 ratio in heart rate and a 1:10,000 ratio in heart weight. On the other hand, not much difference was noted between the duration of the first sound of the pony and man, in spite of a 1:5 difference in heart weight.

Number of Components of the Second Sound. Two components, the aortic and the pulmonic, were found in pony, man, dog, cat, and guinea pig. The fact that only one component was found in the rabbit, rat, and mouse may not have a particular significance because of the difficulty in recording the pulmonary component if the microphone is not close enough to the second left interspace, as it is possible it happened in small animals. This was revealed by the small magnitude of the second heart sound in these animals.

First sound—second sound interval. The interval between first and second sounds represents grossly the duration of ventricular systole. It was 500 msec. in the pony, 350 in man, 204 in the dog, 190 in the cat, 120 in the rabbit and guinea pig, and 50 msec. both in the white rat and the white mouse. Thus, there was a 1:10 ratio in the duration of ventricular systole, inversely equivalent to that of heart rate but certainly not to that of heart weight (grossly 1:100,000).

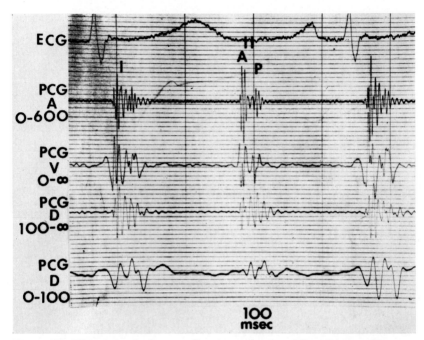

FIGURE 66. Electro- and phonocardiograms of a cat. The phonocardiograms, simultaneously recorded, show the displacement tracing in two bands, and the velocity and acceleration tracings without filtration. The acceleration tracing shows clearly the *a* and *b* components of the first sound.

Most of our findings have an interest chiefly in terms of comparison with pathologic data. However, a few of them have greater significance for the general interpretation of the mechanism of the heart sounds as well as for general physiologic interpretation. The following facts have been ascertained.

1. The heart rate increases from the larger to the small animals without exact correlation with the decrease in size and weight.

2. The *Q-I interval* decreases from the larger to the smaller animals without exact correlation with either heart weight or heart rate as the white mouse had an interval which was about 1/3 that of man.

3. *Components.* The first sound presented three components in the larger animals, only two in the smaller. The second sound presented two components in the larger animals, one in the

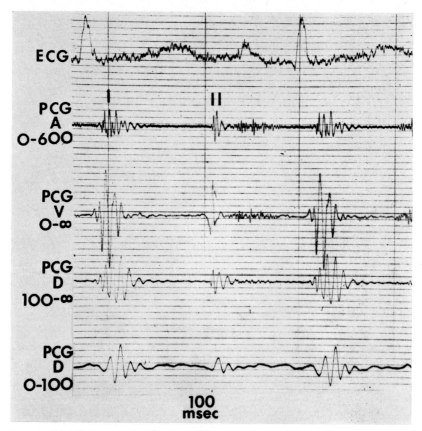

FIGURE 67. Electro- and phonocardiogram of a rabbit. The phonocardiograms are from above: acceleration, velocity, and two displacement tracings
(in a high and a low band). The vibrations in diastole are due to respiration.

smaller. If one considers the technical difficulty of recording
heart sounds in small animals, it is likely that small animals have
the same number of components as the larger ones.

4. *Duration of Ventricular Systole.* A 1:10 ratio between
smaller and larger animals was found, which correlated well with
the inverse ratio of the heart rates.

5. *Interval Between a and b Components of the First Heart
Sound.* This interval was longer in larger animals, shorter in
smaller animals. It was found to be about the same in the cat,
rabbit, and smaller laboratory animals. Studies from our group

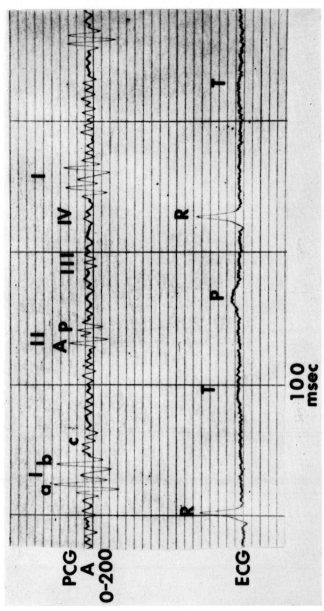

FIGURE 68. Electro- and phonocardiogram of a guinea pig. The phonocardiogram is an acceleration tracing in the band 0-200 Hz and clearly shows the *a*
and *b* components of the first sound, the *A* and *P* components of the second
sound, and the third sound.

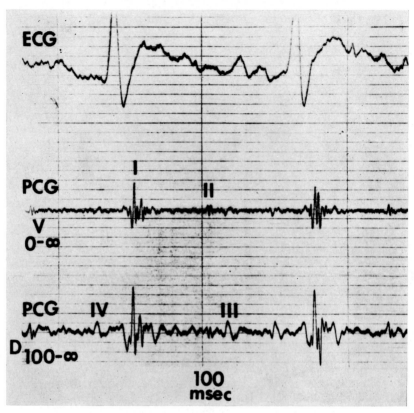

FIGURE 69. Electro- and phonocardiograms of a white rat. From above:
velocity and displacement phonocardiograms. The last tracing reveals the
third and fourth sounds.

have demonstrated that both components originate in the left
ventricle, that the first of them is only in part (10%) related to
mitral valve tension, and that both seem related to waves of
acceleration and deceleration between the apex and base of the
left ventricle. The interval between them is probably determined
by the length of the ventricle, the rapidity of contraction, and
the duration of the isovolumic tension period, the latter being
largely dependent about the level of aortic pressure. The inter-
relation between these factors may explain the relative slow decrease in this interval between large and small animals. The
rapidity of contraction probably increases from the larger to the

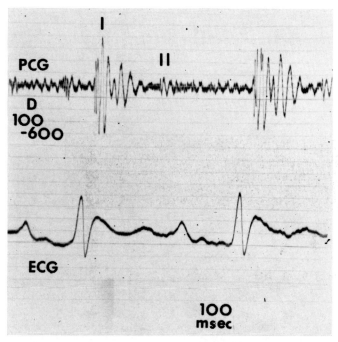

FIGURE 70. Electro- and phonocardiogram of a white mouse. The first sound is split in two (*a* and *b* components). The second sound is small.

smaller animals; the aortic pressure has only a minor decrease in this series; the size of the ventricle, on the contrary has an enormous decrease. This would point out to the relatively lesser importance of left ventricular size in comparison to the other factors.

Guinea pigs and rabbits frequently have respiratory murmurs superimposed over the cardiac sounds because of grossly similar cardiac and respiratory rates.

Murmurs caused by valvular damage are clearly recognizable and tend to be low-pitched and musical in large animals. Innocent murmurs are frequently found in the horse (Niemetz, Reisinger, Detweiler, 1961).

Bibliography

Agress, C. M., and Fields, L. G.: New method for analyzing heart vibrations. I. Low frequency vibrations. Am. J. Cardiol., 4:184, 1959.

Agress, C. M., Fields, L. G., Wegner, S., Wilburne, M., Schichman, M.D. and Muller, R. M.: The normal vibrocardiogram; physiologic variations and relation to cardiodynamic events. Am. J. Cardiol., 8:22, 1961.

Aravanis, C., Feigen, L. P., and Luisada, A. A.: The duration and intervals of normal heart sounds in man. Amer. Heart J., in press, 1971.

Aravanis, C., and Harris, R.: The normal phonocardiogram of the aged. Dis. Chest, 33:214, 1958.

Arevalo, F., and Sakamoto, T.: On the duration of the isovolumetric relaxation period (IVRP) in dog and man. Am. Heart J., 67:651, 1964.

Arevalo, F., Meyer, E. C., MacCanon, D. M., and Luisada, A. A.: Hemodynamic correlates of the third heart sound. J. Appl. Physiol., 207:319, 1964.

Aygen, M. M., and Braunwald, E.: The splitting of the second heart sound in normal subjects and in patients with congenital heart disease. Circulation, 25:328, 1962.

Barlow, J. B., and Shillingford, J.: The use of amyl nitrite in differentiating mitral and aortic systolic murmurs. Brit. Heart J. 29:162, 1958.

Barritt, D. W., and Davies, D. H.: Direct recording of sounds and pressures within the heart. Brit. Heart J., 25:549, 1963.

Battaerd, P. J. T. A.: Further graphic researches on the acoustic phenomena of the heart in normal and pathological conditions. Heart, 6:121, 1915.

Beck, W., Schrire, V., Vogelpoel, L., Nellen, M. and Swanepoel, A.: Hemodynamic effects of amyl nitrite and phenylephrine on the normal human circulation and their relation to changes in cardiac murmurs. Am. J. Cardiol., 8:341, 1961.

Benchimol, A., and Dimond, E. G.: The normal and abnormal apexcardiogram; its physiologic variation and its relation to intracardiac events. Am. J. Cardiol., 12:368, 1963.

Benchimol, A., Dimond, E. G., and Carson, J. C.: The value of the apexcardiogram as a reference tracing in phonocardiography. Am. Heart J., 61:485, 1961.

Beranek, L. L.: Acoustic Measurements. New York, 1949, John Wiley & Sons, Inc.

Bernstein, J. G. M., and Luisada, A. A.: A quantitative study of the phonocardiogram in normal young adults. Livro Jubilar do Prof. E. Coelho. Sebastian Rodrigues, Lisbon, 1966 (p. 179).

249

Beruti, J. A.: Fernauskultation und Registrierung der fötalen Herztöne, Arch. f. Gynäk. *132*:52, 1927.

Bethel, C. S., and Crow, E. W.: Heart sounds in the aged. Am. J. Cardiol., *11*:763, 1963.

Bianchi, A.: *The phoendoscope and its practical application* (translated from Italian by A. G. Baker). Philadelphia, 1898, Pilling & Son.

Blumberger, K.: Die Untersuchung der Dynamik des Herzens beim Menschen. Ihre Anwendung als Herzleistungsprufüng. Ergebn. inn. med. u. Kinderh., *62*:424, 1942.

Boyer, N. H.: Studies on the third heart sound. Am. Heart J., *23*:797, 1942.

Brandt, J. L., Caccese, A., Dock, W., and Schrager, A.: The motion of the thorax during the heart cycle: a comparison of longitudinal, lateral and dorsoventral ballistocardiograms. J. Clin. Invest. *30*:971, 1951.

Braunwald, E., Moscovitz, H. L., Amram, S. S., Lasser, R. P., Sapin, S. O., Himelstein, A., Ravitch, M. M., and Gordon, A. J.: The hemodynamics of the left side of the heart as studied by simultaneous left atrial, left ventricular and aortic pressures; particular reference to mitral stenosis. Circulation, *12*:69, 1955.

Braunwald, E., Moscovitz, H. L., Amram, S. S., Lasser, R. P., Sapin, S. O., Himmelstein, A., Ravitch, M. M., and Gordon, A. J.: Timing of electrical and mechanical events of the left side of the human heart. J. Appl. Physiol., *8*:309 1955A.

Braunwald, E., Fishman, A. P., and Cournand, A.: Time relationship of dynamic events in the cardiac chambers, pulmonary artery and aorta in man. Circulation Res., *4*:100, 1956.

Brecher, G. A.: Experimental evidence of ventricular diastolic suction. Circulation Res., *4*:513, 1956.

Brecher, G. A., and Kissen, A. T.: Ventricular diastolic suction at normal arterial pressures. Circulation Res., *6*:100, 1958.

Bressou, M.: *L'Electrocardiogramme et le phonocardiogramme du cheval normal.* Paris, 1944, Foudon.

Bruns, D. L.: A general theory of the causes of murmurs in the cardiovascular system. Am. J. Med., *27*:360 1959.

Burch, C. R., and Stock, J. P. P.: A new diaphragmatic stethoscope. Brit. Heart J. *23*:447, 1961.

Butterworth, J. S., Chassin, M. R., and McGrath, R.: *Cardiac Auscultation Including Audio-visual Principles,* ed. 2, New York, 1960, Grune & Stratton, Inc.

Cabot R. C., and Dodge, H. F.: Frequency characteristics of heart and lung sounds. J.A.M.A., *84*:1793, 1925.

Caceres, Cesar A., and Perry, Lowell W.: *The Innocent Murmur.* Little, Brown & Co., 1967.

Calo, A. A.: *Atlas de phonocardiographie clinique.* Paris, 1938, Masson & Cie.

Calo, A. A.: Il quinto tono cardiaco, Cuore e circolaz., *33*:208, 1949.

Calo, A. A.: *Les bruits du Coeur et des Vaisseaux.* Paris, 1950, Masson & Cie.

Caniggia, A., and Bertelli, G.: Fonocardiografia ad alta velocitá: analisi delle vibrazioni componenti i toni ed i soffi cardiaci. Minerva Cardioangiol., *8*:249, 1960.

Carral, R.: *Semiologia Cardiovascular,* ed. 5, Mexico, 1963, Editorial Interamericana, S.A.

Castle, R. F., and Jones, K. L.: The mechanism of respiratory variation in splitting of the second heart sound. Circulation, *24*:180, 1961.

Charton, A., Minot, G., and Bressou, M.: Phonocardiographic study of the normal heart sounds in the horse. Vet. Bull., *15*:54, 1945.

Coermann, R. R., Ziegenruecker, G. H., Wittwer, A. L., and Von Gierke, H. E.: The passive dynamic mechanical properties of the human thorax-abdomen system and of the whole body system. Aerospace Med., *31*:443, 1960.

Cossio, P., and Braun-Menéndez, E.: Desdoblamiento fisiológico de los ruidos del corazón. Rev. argent, cardiol., *2*:149, 1935.

Counihan, T., Messer, A. L., Rappaport, M. B., and Sprague, H. B.: The initial vibrations of the first heart sound. Circulation, *3*:730, 1951.

Craige, E., and Harned, H. S., Jr.: Phonocardiographic and electrocardiographic studies in normal newborn infants. Am. Heart J., *65*:180, 1963.

Crevasse, L.: The use of a vasopressor agent as a diagnostic aid in auscultation. Am. Heart J., *58*:821, 1959.

Crevasse, L., Wheat, M. W., Wilson, J. R., Leeds, R. F., and Taylor, W. J.: The mechanism of the generation of the third and fourth heart sounds. Circulation, *25*:635, 1962.

Detweiler, D. K.: The heart. In Hoskins, H. P., Lacroix, J. V., and Mayer, K., editors: *Canine Medicine,* ed. 2. Santa Barbara, 1959, American Veterinary Publications, Inc.

Detweiler, D. K., and Patterson, D. F.: Abnormal heart sounds and murmurs of the dog. J. Small Anim. Pract., *8*:193, 1967.

DiBartolo, G., Nunez-Dey, D., Muiesan, G., MacCanon, D. M., and Luisada, A. A.: Hemodynamic correlates of the first heart sound. Am. J. Physiol., *201*:888, 1961.

Dock, W.: Mode of production of the first heart sound. Arch. Int. Med., *51*:737, 1933.

Dock, W.: The forces needed to evoke sounds from cardiac tissues, and the attention of heart sounds. Circulation, *19*:376, 1959.

Dock, W., Grandell, F., and Taubman, F.: The physiologic third heart sound: its mechanism and relation to protodiastolic gallop. Am. Heart J., *50*:449, 1955.

Dressler, W.: *Die Brustwandpulsationen als Symptome von Herz- und Gefässkrankheiten.* Vienna, 1933, Wilhelm Maudrich.

Dukes, H. H.: *The Physiology of Domestic Animals,* ed. 6, Ithaca, N.Y., 1947, Comstock Pub. Assoc.

Dunn, F. L.: Absolute vs. acoustic standardization in electrostethography and the need for studying cardiac vibrations as transients. IRE Tr. M. Electron. PGME-*6*:17, 1957.

Dunn, F. L., and Rahm, W. E., Jr.: Electrostethography. II. New method for study of precordial transmission of cardiodynamics. Am. Heart J., *44*:95, 1952.

Dunn, F. L., and Rahm, W. E., Jr.: Electrostethography. III. Crystal microphone characteristics at low frequencies for the study of cardiodynamics. Am. Heart J., *45*:519, 1953.

Dunn, F. L., and Rahm, W. E., Jr.: The problem of calibration in heart sound recording. Am. Heart J., *46*:237, 1953A.

Ebina, T., Kanagarni, H., Katsura, T., Tanaka, N., Kikuchi, Y., and Okuyama, D.: An analysis of the frequency spectrum with sound spectrography. Lung (Tokyo) *9*:64, 1962.

Eddleman, E. E., Jr., and Willis, K.: The kinetocardiogram. III. The distribution of forces over the anterior chest. Circulation, *8*:569, 1953.

Eddleman, E. E., Jr., Willis, K., Reeves, T. J., and Harrison, T. R.: The kinetocardiogram. I. Method of recording precordial movements. Circulation, *8*:269, 1953.

Eddleman, E. E., Jr., Willis, K., Christianson, L., Pierce, J. R., and Walker, R. P.: The kinetocardiogram. II. The normal configuration and amplitude. Circulation, *8*:370, 1953A.

Faber, J. J.: Damping of sound on the chest surface. Circulation Res., *13*:352, 1963.

Faber, J. J.: Origin and conduction of the mitral sound in the heart. Circulation Res., *14*:426, 1964.

Faber, J. J., and Burton, A. C.: Spread of heart sounds over chest wall. Circulation Res., *11*:96, 1962.

Faber, J. J., ond Purvis, J. H.: Conduction of cardiovascular sound along arteries. Circulation Res., *12*:308, 1963.

Feruglio, G. A.: Intracardiac phonocardiography: A valuable diagnostic technique in congenital and acquired heart disease. Am. Heart J., *58*:827, 1959.

Feruglio, G. A.: An intracardiac sound generator for the study of the transmission of heart murmurs in man. Am. Heart J., *63*:232, 1962A.

Feruglio, G. A.: A new method for producing, calibrating, and recording intracardiac sounds in man. Am. Heart J., *65*:377, 1963.

Feruglio, G. A.: *Intracardiac Auscultation and Phonocardiography*. Torino, 1964, Edizioni Mineiva Medica.

Feruglio, G. A., Dalla Volta, S., Lewis, D. H., and Wallace, J. D.: La phonocardiographie intracardiaque chez l'homme. Arch. mal coeur, *52*:1156, 1959.

Fishleder, B. L.: Las fases del ciclo cardiaco. Su estudio grafico y su valor clinico. Princ. cardiol., *6*:123, 1959.

Fishleder, B. L.: Fonocardiografía fetal. Princ. cardiol., *7*:59, 1960.

Fishleder, B. L.: La Prueba de Valsalva en fonocardiografia clinica. Fourth World Congress of Cardiology, Mexico, vol. I-B, 1963, p. 428.

Fletcher, H.: *Speech and Hearing in Communication*. New York, 1953, D. Van Nostrand Co., Inc.

Fletcher, H., and Munson, W. A.: Loudness, its definition, measurement, and claculation. J. Acoust. Soc. Am., *5*:82, 1933.

Foulger, J. H., Smith, P. E., Jr., and Fleming, A. J.: Changes in cardiac vibrational intensity in response to physiologic stress. Am. Heart J., *34*:507, 1947.

Foulger, J. H., Smith, P. E., Jr., and Fleming, A. J.: Cardiac vibrational intensity and cardiac output. Am. Heart J., *35*:953, 1948.

Frank, O.: Die unmittelbare Registrierung der Herztoene. Münch. med Wchnschr., *51*:953, 1904.

Frederick, H. A., and Dodge, H. F.: The stethophone, an electrical stethoscope. Bell System Techn. J., *3*:351, 1924.

Friedman, S., Robie, W. A., and Harris, T. N.: Occurrence of innocent adventitious cardiac sounds in childhood. Pediatrics, *4*:782, 1949.

Geckeler, G. D., Likoff, W., Mason, D., Riesz, R. R., and Wirth, C. H.: Cardiospectrograms. A Preliminary report. Am. Heart J., *48*:189, 1954.

Gleason, W. L., and Braunwald, E.: Studies on the first derivative of the ventricular pressure pulse in man. J. Clin. Invest., *41*:80, 1962.

Gmachl, E.: Ueber die Amplitude des ersten Herztones. Vehhandl. Deut. Ges. Kreislaufforsch., *20*:375, 1954.

Gmachl, E.: Zum Problem der Enstehung des ersten Herztones. L. Kreislaufforsch, *41*:512, 1952.

Goldman, S.: *Frequency Analysis, Modulation and Noise.* New York, 1948, McGraw-Hill Book Co., Inc.

Grayzel, J.: Gallop rhythm of the heart. Circulation, *20*:703, 1959 (Abst.).

Grayzel, J.: Gallop rhythm of the heart. I. Atrial gallop, ventricular gallop and systolic sounds. Am. J. Med., *28*:578, 1960.

Grayzel, J.: Gallop rhythm of the heart. II. Quadruple rhythm and its relation to summation and augmented gallops. Circulation, *20*:1053, 1959A.

Grishman, A., Bleifer, S. B., and Donoso, E.: Clinical phonocardiography. Graphic analysis of clinical auscultation. Advances Int. Med., *10*:179, 1960.

Groedel, F. M., and Miller, M.: Intratracheal auscultation. Exper. Med. & Surg., *8*:42, 1950.

Groom, D.: The effect of background noise on cardiac auscultation. Am. Heart J., *52*:781, 1956.

Groom, D., and Boone, J. A.: The recording of heart sounds and vibrations. II. The application of an electronic pickup in the graphic recording of subaudible and audible frequencies. Exper. Med. & Surg., *14*:255, 1956.

Groom, D., and Sihvonen, Y. T.: High sensitivity capacitance pickup for heart sounds and murmurs. IRE Tr. M. Electron. PGME- *9*:35, 1957.

Groom, D., Underwood, A. F., Bidwell, J. B., and Lindberg, E.: The recording of heart sounds and vibrations. I. Historical review and description of a new electronic direct-contact vibration pickup. Exper. Med. & Surg., *14*:239, 1956.

Groom, D., Chapman, W., Francis, W. W., Bass, A., and Sihvonen, Y. T.: The normal systolic murmur. Ann. Int. Med., *52*:134, 1960.

Guenther, K. H.: *Comparative Extracardiac and Intracardiac Phonocardiography.* Berlin, Akademie-Verlag, 1969.

Gupta, P. D., Sainani, G. S., and Luisada, A. A.: Comparison between the Valsalva maneuver and a newly-devised expiratory valve on splitting of the second heart sound. Dis. Chest, *51*:603, 1967.

Hamlin, R. L., Robinson, F. R., Smith, C. R. and Marsland, W. P.: Heart sounds of healthy Macaca mulatta. J. Appl. Physiol., *17*:199, 1962.

Hamlin, R. L., Smetzer, D. L., and Smith, C. R.: The electrocardiogram, phonocardiogram, and derived ventricular activation process of domestic cats. Am. J. Vet. Res., *24*:792, 1963.

Harvey, W. P.: Technique and art of auscultation. *In* Segal, B. L., editor: *The Theory and Practice of Auscultation.* Philadelphia, 1964, F. A. Davis Co., p. 50.

Harvey, W. P.: Abnormalities of the first and second heart sounds in the diagnosis of heart disease. *In* Segal, B. L., editor: *The Theory and Practice of Auscultation.* Philadelphia, 1964, F. A. Davis Co., p. 117A.

Heintzen, P.: *Quantitative Phonokardiographie.* Stuttgart, 1960, Georg Thieme Verlag.

Heintzen, P., and Vietor, K. W.: The diacardiac phonogram. Am. Heart J., *65*:59, 1963.

Henderson, A. A., Brutsaert, D. L., Parmley, W. W., and Sonnenblick, E. H.: Myocardial mechanics in papillary muscles of the rat and cat. Am. J. Physiol., *217*:1273, 1969.

Hess, W. R.: Die graphische Aufzeichnung der Herstöne nach neueren Methoden. Pflüger's Arch. Physiol., *180*:35, 1920.

Holldack, K.: Die Phonokardiographie, ihre Bedeutung für die sinnesphysiologischen Grundlagen der Herzauskultation und ihre diagnostische Verwendung.

254 SOUNDS OF THE NORMAL HEART

Ergebn. inn. Med. u. Kinderh., *3*:407, 1952.

Holldack, K., and Bayer, O.: Phonokardiographische Untersuchungen bei Mitral-stenosen nach Kommissurotomie. Stschr. Kreislaufforsch., *42*:721, 1953.

Holldack, K., and Wolf, D.: *Atlas und kurzgefasstes Lehrbuch der Phonokardio-graphie and verwandter Untersuchungsmethoden.* Stuttgart, 1956, Georg Thieme Verlag.

Holldack, K., Luisada, A. A., and Ueda, H.: Standardization of phonocardiography. Am. J. Cardiol., *15*:419, 1965.

Hollis, W. J., and Vidrine, A.: Time relations of the subaudible low-frequency precordial thrust-impacts and electromechanical events of cardiac contraction and systolic ejection. Exper. Med. & Surg. *17*:234, 1959.

Hurst, J. W.: Some comments on auscultation of the heart. I. The intensity of the first heart sound at the apex. J.M.A. Georgia, *46*:47, 1957.

Jacono, A., and Friedland, C.: Frequency characteristics of extra sounds. Am. J. Cardiol., *4*:207, 1959.

Johnston, F. D., and Overy, D. C.: Vibrations of low frequency over the pre-cordium. Circulation, *3*:579, 1951.

Krol, B., and Luisada, A. A.: Amplitud del segundo ruido cardiaco en la base del corazón. Prensa Med. Argentina, *53*:578, 1966.

Landes, G.: Über Brustkorbschwingungen bei der Herzaktion, Deutsches Arch. klin Med., *186*:288, 1940.

Landes, G.: Neure Untersuchungen über Herzstoss und Brustwandpulsation. Deutsches Arch. klin. Med., *188*:403, 1942.

Laurens, P.: Considérations sûr l'origine des bruits du coeur. Actual Cardiovasc. Medico-Chir., 4th series, 104, 1968.

Leatham, A.: Phonocardiography. Brit. M. Bull., *8*:333, 1952.

Leatham, A.: Splitting of the first and second heart sounds. Lancet, *2*:607, 1954.

Leatham, A.: Auscultation of the heart. Lancet, *2*:703, 757, 1958.

Leatham, A.: The value of auscultation in cardiology, Arch. Int. Med, *105*:349, 1960.

Leatham, A., and Towers, M.: Splitting of the second heart sound in health. Brit. Heart J., *13*:575, 1951.

Leatham, A., Segal, B., and Shafter, H.: Auscultatory and phonocardiographic findings in healthy children with systolic murmurs. Brit. Heart J., *25*:451, 1963.

Levin, H. S., Runco, V., Wooley, C. F., Goodwin, R. S., and Ryan, J. M.: The effect of respiration on cardiac murmurs. An auscultatory illusion. Am. J. Med., *33*:236, 1962.

Levine, S. A., and Harvey, W. P.: *Clinical Auscultation of the Heart,* ed. 2. Phil-adelphia, 1959. W. B. Saunders Co.

Levine, S. A., and Likoff, W. B.: Some notes on the transmission of heart murmurs. Ann. Int. Med., *21*:298, 1944.

Lewis, D. H.: The nature of sound and the principles governing its transmission. *In* Segal, B. L. editor: *The Theory and Practice of Auscultation.* Philadelphia, 1964, F. A. Davis Co.

Lewis, D. H., Deitz, G. W., Wallace, J. D., and Brown, J. R., Jr.: Intracardiac phonocardiography in man. Circulation, *16*:764, 1957.

Lewis, D. H., Deitz, G. W., Wallace, J. D., and Brown, J. R. Jr.: Intracardiac phono-cardiography. IRE Tr. M. Electron. PGME- *9*:31, 1957A.

Lewis, J. K., and Dock, W.: The origin of the heart sounds and their variations in myocardial disease. J.A.M.A., *110*:271, 1938.

Lewis, T.: *The Mechanism and Graphic Registration of the Heart Beat.* London, 1925, Shaw & Sons.

Lian, C., and Golblin, V.: Les bruits du coeur foetal in utero (étude phonocardiographique). Arch. mal coeur, *31*:173, 1938.

Lian, C., Milnot, G., and Welti, J. J.: *Phonocardiographie. Auscultation collective.* Paris, 1941, Masson & Cie.

Luisada, A. A.: Les foyers d'auscultation du thorax. Coeur et Méd. Int., *8*:3, 1969.

Luisada, A. A.: Occurrence and cause of an auricular sound in the horse. Vet. Med., *36*:5, 1941A.

Luisada, A. A.: Phonocardiographie éxpérimentale Actual. Cardiovasc. Medio-Chirurg., Paris, Masson, 1968, p. 91.

Luisada, A. A.: The diastolic sounds of the heart in normal and pathological conditions. Acta med. scandinav., *142*:685 (supp. 266), 1952.

Luisada, A. A.: *The Heart Beat.* New York, 1953, Paul B. Hoeber, Inc., Medical Book Dept. of Harper & Row, Publishers, Inc.

Luisada, A. A.: The expanding horizon of phonocardiography. Arch. Kreislaufforsch., *33*:38, 1960.

Luisada, A. A.: *From Auscultation to Phonocardiography.* St. Louis, 1965, Mosby.

Luisada, A. A., and Cortis, B.: The dynamic events of the normal heart in man. Acta. Cardiol., *25*:203, 1970.

Luisada, A. A., and Di Bartolo, G.: High frequency phonocardiography. Am. J. Cardiol., *8*:51, 1961.

Luisada, A. A., and Gamma, G.: Clinical calibration in phonocardiography. Am. Heart J., *48*:826, 1954.

Luisada, A. A., Gagnon, G., and Ikeda, H.: The first heart sound and the dynamic events in ventricular ectopic beats and in paced beats. Am. J. Cardiol., *25*:529, 1970.

Luisada, A. A., Kurz, H., Slodki, S. J., MacCanon, D. M., and Krol, B.: Normal first sounds with nonfunctional tricuspid valve or right ventricle: clinical and experimental evidence. Circulation, *35*:119, 1967.

Luisada, A. A., and Liu, C. K.: Simple methods for recording intracardiac electrocardiograms and phonocardiograms during left or right heart catheterization. Am. Heart J., *54*:531, 1957.

Luisada, A. A., Liu, C. K.: *Intracardiac Phenomena in Right and Left Heart Catheterization.* New York, 1958A, Grune & Stratton, Inc.

Luisada, A. A., and MacCanon, D. M.: The phases of the cardiac cycle. Am. Heart J., 1971 (in press).

Luisada, A. A., MacCanon, D. M., Bruce, D. W., Worthen, M., Argano, B., Siwadlowski, W., and Kurz, H.: Heart sounds of the right heart. J. Appl. Physiol., *25*:362, 1968.

Luisada, A. A., and Magri, G.: The low frequency tracings of the precordium and epigastrium in normal subjects and cardiac patients. Am. Heart J., *44*:545, 1952.

Luisada, A. A., and Mautner, H.: Experimental studies on functional murmurs and extra-sounds of the heart. Exper. Med. & Surg., *1*:282, 1943.

Luisada, A. A., and Pérez Montes, L.: A phonocardiographic study of apical diastolic murmurs simulating those of mitral stenosis. Ann. Int. Med., *33*:56, 1950.

Luisada, A. A., and Shah, P. M.: Controversial and changing aspects of auscultation. I. Areas of auscultation: a new concept. II. Normal and abnormal first and second sounds. Am. J. Cardiol., *11*:774, 1963.

Luisada, A. A., and Shah, P. M.: Controversial changing aspects of auscultation. III. Diastolic sounds. IV. Intervals. V. Systolic sounds. Am. J. Cardiol., *13*:243, 1964.

Luisada, A. A., and Zalter, R.: Phonocardiography. III. Design of the ideal phonocardiograph. Am. J. Cardiol., *4*:24, 1959.

Luisada, A. A., and Zalter, R.: A new standardized and calibrated phonocardiographic system. IRE Tr. M. Electron. PGME- 7:15, 1960.

Luisada, A. A., Weisz, L., and Hantman, H. W.: A comparative study of electrocardiogram and heart sounds in common and domestic mammals. Cardiologia (Basel), *8*:63, 1944.

Luisada, A. A., Mendoza, F., and Alimurung, M. M.: The duration of normal heart sounds. Brit. Heart J., *11*:41, 1949.

Luisada, A. A., Haring, O. M., and Zilli, A. B.: Apical diastolic murmurs simulating mitral stenosis. II. Graphic differentiation. Ann. Int. Med., *42*:644, 1955.

Luisada, A. A., Richmond, L., and Aravanis, C.: Selective phonocardiography. Am. Heart J., *51*:221, 1956.

Luisada, A. A., Liu, C. K., Aravanis, C., and Testelli, M.: Intracardiac vibrations of sonic frequency within the right and left hearts. Acta cardiol., *13*:338, 1958A.

Luisada, A. A., Liu, C. K., Aravanis, C., Testelli, M., and Morris, J.: On the mechanism of production of the heart sounds. Am. Heart J., *55*:383, 1958B.

Luisada, A. A., Inoue, T., and Katz, M.: On the amplitude and duration of the precordial vibrations of normal man. Cardiologia (Basel), *42*:273, 1963.

Luisada, A. A., Liu, C. K., Szatkowski, J., and Slodki, S. J.: Intracardiac phonocardiography in 172 cases studied by left or right heart catheterization or both. Acta cardiol., *18*:533, 1964.

Luisada, A. A., and Sainani, G. S.: *A Primer of Cardia Diagnosis.* W. Green, St. Louis, 1968.

Maass, H., and Weber, A.: Herzschallregistrierung mittels differenzierender Filter: Eine Studie zur Herzschallnormung. Cardiologia (Basel), *21*:773, 1952.

MacCanon, D. M., Arevalo, F., and Meyer, E. C.: Direct detection and timing of aortic valve closure. Circulation Res., *14*:387, 1964.

MacCanon, D. M., Bruce, D. W., Lynch, P. R., and Nickerson, J. L.: Mass excursion parameters of first heart sound energy. J. Appl. Physiol., *27*:649, 1969.

McDonald, D. A.: Murmurs in relation to turbulence and eddy formation in the circulation. Circulation, *16*:278, 1957.

McGregor, M., Rappaport, M. B., Sprague, H. B., and Friedlich, A. L.: The calibration of heart sound intensity. Circulation, *13*:252, 1956.

McKee, M. H.: Heart sounds in normal children. Am. Heart J., *16*:79, 1938.

McKusick, V. A.: *Cardiovascular Sound in Health and Disease.* Baltimore, 1958, Williams & Wilkins Co.

McKusick, V. A.: Musical murmurs: spectral phonocardiographic studies. *In* Segal, B. L., (ed.): *The Theory and Practice of Auscultation.* Philadelphia, 1964, F. A. Davis Co., p. 93.

McKusick, V. A., Talbot, S. A., and Webb, G. N.: Spectral phonocardiography; problems and prospects in the application of the Bell sound spectograph to phonocardiography. Bull Johns Hopkins Hosp., *94*:187, 1954.

Magri, G., Jona, E., Messina, D., and Actis-Dato, A.: Direct recording of heart sounds and murmurs from the epicardial surface of the exposed human heart. Am. Heart J., 57:449, 1959.

Magri, G., Jona, E., Gamna, G., Messina, D., and Guglielmini, G.: Il fonocardiogramma epicardico dell'uomo. I. Nella stenosi mitralica, Minerva med., 49:36, 1958.

Mannheimer, E.: Calibrated phonocardiography. A new technique for clinical use. Am. Heart J., 21:151, 1951.

Mannheimer, E.: Phonocardiography in children. Advances Pediat., 7:171, 1955.

Mannheimer, E.: Standardization of phonocardiography. Am. Heart J., 54:214, 1957.

Marey, E. J.: La méthode graphique dans les sciences expérimentales at principalement en physiologie et en médecine, ed. 2. Paris, 1885, Masson & Cie.

Meisner, J. E., and Rushmer, R. F.: Production of sounds in distensible tubes. Circulation Res., 12:651, 1963A.

Miller, A., and White, P. D.: Crystal microphone for pulse wave recording. Am. Heart J., 21:504, 1941.

Mills, J.: Sound. In Glasser, O., (ed.) : Medical Physics, vol. 1. Chicago, 1944, Year Book Medical Publishers, Inc., p. 1438.

Mori, M., Shah, P. M., MacCanon, D. M., and Luisada, A. A.: Hemodynamic correlates of the various components of the second heart sound. Cardiologia (Basel) , 44:65, 1964.

Moscovitz, H. L., and Wilder, A. J.: Pressure events of the cardiac cycle in the dog. Normal right and left heart. Circulation Res., 4:574, 1956.

Moscovitz, H. L., Donoso, E., Gelb, I. J., and Welkowitz, W.: Intracardiac phonocardiography. Correlation of mechanical, acoustic and electric events of the cardiac cycle. Circulation, 18:983, 1958.

Mounsey, P.: Precordial pulsations in relation to cardiac movement and sounds. Brit. Heart J., 21:457, 1959.

Muiesan, G., MacCanon, D. M., Nuñez-Dey, D., and Di Bartolo, G.: Hemodynamic correlates of the fourth heart sound. Am. J. Physiol., 201:1090, 1961.

Neumann-Kleinpaul, K., and Steffan, H.: Zur graphischen Darstellung der Herztöne bei Tier und Mensch. Arch. Tierheilk. 65:629, 1932.

Neumann-Kleinpaul, K., and Steffan, H.: Die kombinierte Elektrokardiogramm-herztonaufnahme bei Tier und Mensch. Arch. Tierheilk., 66:1, 1933.

Oberhoffer, G.: Zur Methodik der Frequenzanalyse der Herztöne, Verhandl. deutsch. Ges. Kreislaufforsch., 20:369, 1954.

Ohm, R.: Der sogenannte dritte Herzton und seine Beziehungen zur diastolischen Kammerfullüng. Berl. klin. Wchnschr., 58:600, 1921.

Ongley, P. A., Sprague, H. B., Rappaport, M. B., and Nadas, A. S.: Heart Sounds and Murmurs. New York, 1960, Grune & Stratton, Inc.

Orias, O., and Braun-Menéndez, E.: The Heart Sounds in Normal and Pathological Conditions. London, 1939, Oxford University Press.

Patterson, D. F., Detweiler, D. K., and Glendenning, S. A.: Heart sounds and murmurs of the normal horse. N. Y. Acad. Sci., 127:242, 1965.

Perloff, J. K., and Harvey, W. P.: Mechanisms of fixed splitting of the second heart sound. Circulation, 18:998, 1958A.

Piemme, T. E., and Dexter, L.: High frequency events of the cardiac cycle. Fed. Proc. 22:642, 1963 (Abst.) .

Piemme, T. E., Barnett, G. O. and Dexter, C.: Relationship of heart sounds to acceleration of blood flow. Circul. Res., 18:303, 1966.

Pintor, P., Gamna, G., Dughera, L., and Magri, G.: II fonocardiogramma esofageo normale, Minerva med., *49*:33, 1958.

Potain, P. C. E.: Note sur les dédoublements normaux des bruits du coeur. Bull et mém. Soc. méd. hôp. Paris, *3*:138, 1866.

Priola, D. V., Osadjan, C. E., and Randall, W. C.: Functional characteristics of the ventricular inflow and outflow tracts. Fed. Proc., *23*:463, 1954.

Randall, J. E.: *Elements of Biophysics.* Year Book Publ. Co., Inc., Chicago, 1958.

Rappaport, M. B., and Sprague, H. B.: Physiologic and physical laws that govern auscultation and their clinical application. The acoustic stethoscope and the electrical amplifying stethoscope and stethography. Am. Heart J., *21*:257, 1941.

Rappaport, M. B., and Sprague, H. B.: The graphic registration of the normal heart sounds. Am. Heart J., *23*:591, 1942.

Rappaport, M. B., and Sprague, H. B.: The effects of tubing bore on stethoscope efficiency. Am. Heart J., *42*:605, 1951.

Ravin, A.: *Auscultation of the Heart.* Chicago, Year Book Medical Publishers, Inc., 1958.

Reeves, T. J., Hefner, L. L., Jones, W. B., Coghlan, C., Prieto, G., and Carroll, J.: The hemodynamic determinants of the rate of change in pressure in the left ventricle during isometric contraction. Am. Heart J., *60*:745, 1960.

Reynolds, O.: An experimental investigation of the circumstances which determine whether the motion of water shall be direct or sinuous, and of the law of resistance in parallel channels. Philos. Tr. Roy. Soc. London, *174*:935, 1883.

Richards, A. G., Simonson, E., and Visscher, M. B.: Electrocardiogram and phonocardiogram of adult and newborn mice in normal conditions and under the effect of cooling, hypoxia and potassium. Am. J. Physiol., *174*:293, 1953.

Rodbard, S.: Flow through collapsible tubes: augmented flow produced by resistance at the outlet. Circulation, *11*:280, 1955.

Rodbard, S.: Transients in heart sounds and murmurs. IRE Tr. M. Electron. PGME-*9*:12, 1957.

Rodbard, S.: The production and physical qualities of sound in the cardiovascular system. In Segal, B. L., (ed.) : *The Theory and Practice of Auscultation.* Philadelphia, 1964, F. A. Davis Co., p. 26.

Rodbard, S., and Saiki, H.: Flow through collapsible tubes. Am. Heart J., *46*:715, 1953.

Rodbard, S., Mendelson, C. E., and Elisberg, E. I.: Vibration analysis of heart sounds and murmurs. Cardiologia (Basel) , *27*:144, 1955.

Rosa, L. M.: The "displacement" vibrocardiogram of the precordium in the low frequency range. Am. J. Cardiol., *4*:191, 1959.

Rosa, L. M., and Luisada, A. A.: Low frequency tracings of precordial displacement and acceleration. Technical comparison of various systems. Am. J. Cardiol., *4*:669, 1959.

Rouanet, J.: Analyse des bruits du coeur. Thesis no. 592, Paris, 1832.

Safonov, Y. D.: The biohydraulic mechanism producing heart sounds. Cor et Vasa, *10*:295, 1968.

Sainani, G. S., Bruce, D. W., MacCanon, D. M., and Luisada, A. A.: Respiratory alterations of the components of the first heart sound. Cardiologia, *52*:252, 1968.

Sainani, G. S., and Luisada, A. A.: "Mapping" of the precordium. I. Heart sounds of normal subjects. Am. J. Cardiol., *19*:788, 1967.

Sakai, A., Feigen, L. P., and Luisada, A. A.: Frequency distribution of the heart sounds in normal man. Cardiovas. Res. (London) (in press, 1971).

Sakamoto, T., Kusukawa, R., MacCanon, D. M., and Luisada, A. A.: Hemodynamic determinants of the amplitude of the first heart sound. Circulation Res., 16:45, 1965.

Shafter, H. A.: Splitting of the second heart sound. Am. J. Cardiol., 6:1013, 1960.

Shah, P. M., and Slodki, S. J.: The Q-II interval: a study of the second heart sound in normal adults and in systemic hypertension. Circulation, 29:551, 1964.

Shah, P. M., and Slodki, S. J.: The duration of the Q-II interval in pulmonary hypertension. CMS Quart., 25:108, 1965.

Shah, P. M., Slodki, S. J., and Luisada, A. A.: A revision of the "classic" areas of auscultation of the heart. A physiologic approach. Am. J. Med., 36:293, 1964.

Shah, P. M., Slodki, S. J., and Luisada, A. A.: A physiologic concept of auscultation. Acta Cardiol., 19:111, 1964A.

Slodki, S. J., Hussain, A. T., and Luisada, A. A.: The Q-II interval. III. A study of the second heart sound in old age. J. Am. Geriatr. Soc., 17:673, 1969.

Smith, H. L., Essex, H. E., and Baldes, E. J.: Study of movements of heart valves and of heart sounds. Ann. Int. Med., 33:1357, 1950.

Smith, J. R.: Observations on the mechanism of the physiologic third heart sound. Am. Heart J., 28:661, 1944.

Smith, J. R., Edwards, J. C., and Kountz, W. B.: The use of the cathode ray for recording heart sounds and vibrations. III. Total cardiac vibrations in one hundred normal subjects. Am. Heart J., 21:228, 1941.

Smith, J. R., Gilson, A. S., and Kountz, W. B.: The use of the cathode ray for recording heart sounds and vibrations. II. Studies of the muscular element of the first heart sound. Am. Heart J., 21:17, 1941A.

Soloff, L. A., Wilson, M. F., Winters, W. L., Jr., and Zatuchni, J.: Responses of cardiac murmurs to norepinephrine. Circulation, 18:783, 1958 (Abst.).

Soulié, P.: Intracardiac phonocardiography. Presented at World Congress of Cardiology. Washington, D.C., 1954.

Soulié, P., Laurens, P., Bouchard, F., Cornu, C., and Brial, E.: Enregistrement des pressions et des bruits intracardiaques à l'aide d'un micromanomètre. Bull. et mém. Soc. méd. hôp. Paris, 73:713, 1957.

Soulié, P., Baculard, P., Bouchard, F., Cornu, C., Laurens, P., and Wolff, F.: Le cathétérisme due coeur au micromanomètre. Le Son Intracardiaque, Paris, 1961, J. B. Baillière et fils.

Sprague, H. B.: A new combined stethoscope chest piece. J.A.M.A., 86:1909, 1926.

Taquini, A. C.: Exploración del corazón por vía esofágica. Buenos Aires, 1936, El Ateneo.

Ueda, H., Kaito, G., and Sakamoto, T.: Clinical Phonocardiography (Japanese). Tokyo, 1963, Nanzando.

van Bogaert, A., van Genabeek, A., Arnoldy, M., Wauters, J., van der Henst, H., Keirsebelik, M., and Vandael, J.: Contribution à l'étude du premier bruit du coeur normal. Arch. mal. coeur, 55:368, 1962.

van Bogaert, A., van Genabeek, A., Arnold, M., Wauters, J., van der Henst, H., Vandael, J., and Keirsebelik, M.: Influence d'une fuite systolique ventriculaire sur l'intensité du premier bruit du coeur. Application à l'insuffisance mitrale. Arch. mal. coeur, 55:961, 1962A.

Von Gierke, H. E., Transmission of vibratory energy through human body tissue.

Proceedings of the First National Biophysical Conference (Columbus, Ohio, 1957), New Haven, Conn., 1959, Yale Univ. Press p. 647.

Von Gierke, H. E.: Transmission of vibratory energy through human tissue. In Glasser, O. (ed.) : Medical Physics, vol. III, Chicago, 1960, Year Book Medical Publishers, Inc., p. 661.

Von Gierke, H. E., Oestreicher, H. L., Franke, E. K., Parrack, H. O., and von Wittern, W. W.: Physics of vibrations in living tissues. J. Appl. Physiol., 4:886, 1952.

Wallace, J. D., Brown, J. R., Jr., Lewis, D. H., and Deitz, G. W.: Part 1. Phono-catheters: their design and application, IRE Tr. M. Electron. PGME- 9:25, 1957.

Wallace, A. G., Mitchell, J. H., Skinner, N. S., and Sarnoff, S. J.: Duration of the phases of left ventricular systole. Circul. Res., 12:611-619, 1963.

Warembourg, H., and Ducloux, G.: L'apexogramme: application à l'étude des cardiopathies mitrales. Arch. mal, coeur, 56:1359, 1963.

Weber, A.: Herzschallregisterierung. Darmstadt, 1944, Dietrich Steinkopff.

Weber, A.: Die Elektrokardiographic und andere graphische Methoden in der Kreislaufdiagnostik, ed. 4. Berlin, 1949, Springer-Verlag.

Weiss, O., and Joachim, G.: Registrierung von Hertzönen und Herzgeräuschen mittels des Phonoskops und ihre Beziehungen zum Elektrokardiogramm. Ztschr. Klin. Med., 73:240, 1911.

Weissel, W.: Ueber negative und kardiodynamische Einfluesse im Schwingungsbild des ersten Herztones. Wein. Klin. Wochschr., 63:294, 1951.

Weissel, W., and Auinger, W.: Das Verhalten des ersten Herztones beim Menschen unter Nor-adrenalin und Adrenalin. Z. Kreislaufforsch., 40:707, 1951.

Weitz, W.: Studien zur Herzphysiologie und pathologie auf Grund kardiograph-ischer Untersuchungen, Ehgebn. inn. Med. u. Kinderh., 22:402, 1922.

Wiggers, C. J.: Circulation in Health and Disease. Lea & Febiger, Philadelphia. 1915, p. 186.

Wiggers, C. J.: Studies on the consecutive phases of the cardiac cycle. I. The dura-tion of the consecutive phases of the cardiac cycle and the criteria for their precise determination. II. The laws governing the relative duration of ven-tricular systole and diastole. Am. J. Physiol., 56:415, 1921.

Wiggers, C. J., and Dean, A., Jr.: The principles and practice of registering heart sounds by direct methods. Am. J. Med. Sc., 153:666, 1917.

Williams, H. B., and Dodge, H. F.: Analysis of heart sounds. Arch. Int. Med., 38:685, 1926.

Winer, D. E., Perry, L. W., and Caceres, C. A.: Heart sound analysis: A three dimensional approach. Am. J. Cardiol., 16:547, 1965.

Wolferth, C. C., and Margolies, A.: Heart sounds. In Stroud, W. D. (ed.) : Diagnosis and treatment of Cardiovascular Disease, vol. I, ed. 4. Philadelphia, 1950, F. A. Davis Co.

Yamakawa, K.: Intracardiac phonocardiography: Recent observations. Jap. Circu-lation J., 24:932, 1960.

Yamakawa, K., Shionoya, Y., Kitamura, K., Nagi, T., Yamamoto, T., and Ohta, S.: Intracardiac phonocardiography, Tohoku J. Exper. Med., 58:311, 1953.

Yarza Iriarte, J. M., Irarte Ezcurdia, M., Rodriguez de Azura, C., Calderón Sanz, A., and Laso Nunez, J. L.: Valor diagnóstico de la fonocardiografia intracardiaca, Rev. espanola cardiol., *14*:194, 1961.

Zalter, R., and Luisada, A. A.: Technical aspects of phonocardiography. *In* Luisada, A. A. (ed.) : *Cardiology,* vol. II, part 3. New York, 1959, Blakiston Div., McGraw-Hill Book Co., Inc., p. 108.

Zalter, R., Hodara, H., and Luisada, A. A.: Phonocardiography. I. General principles and problems of standardization. Am. J. Cardiol., *4*:3, 1959.

Zalter, R., and Luisada, A. A.: Phonocardiography. II. Appraisal and critical analysis of existing systems. Am. J. Cardiol., *4*:16, 1959A.

Zalter, R., Hardy, H. C., and Luisada, A. A.: Acoustic transmission characteristics of the thorax. J. Appl. Physiol., *18*:428, 1963.

Zakrzewski, T. K., Slodki, S. J., and Luisada, A. A.: The first heart sound in atrial septal defect. Am. Heart J., *78*:476, 1969.

Zinsser, H. F., and Kay, C. F.: The straining procedure as an aid in the anatomic localization of cardiovascular murmurs and sounds. Circulation, *1*:523, 1950.

INDEX